COPING WITH THE **COMMON COLD**

COPING WITH THE **COMMON COLD**

by Wendy Murphy

AND THE EDITORS OF TIME-LIFE BOOKS

LIBRARY OF HEALTH / TIME-LIFE BOOKS / ALEXANDRIA, VIRGINIA

**THE AUTHOR:**
Wendy Murphy brings to this work nearly 25 years' experience as a writer and editor in fields as diverse as paleontology and boating, antiques and home repair. Her previous books include two volumes of the TIME-LIFE Encyclopedia of Gardening: *Japanese Gardening* and *Indoor Gardening Under Light*.

**THE CONSULTANTS**
Dr. David A. J. Tyrrell is Deputy Director of the Clinical Research Centre and Head of the Division of Communicable Diseases in Harrow, England. Since 1962 h has also headed the Common Cold Unit in Salisbury, England, the only facility in the world devoted exclusively to the study of this disease. He is the author of *Common Colds and Related Diseases* and *Interferon and its Clinical Potential*.

Dr. Michael F. Parry is Director of Infectious Diseases at Stamford Hospital in Connecticut and Assistant Clinical Professor of Medicine at Columbia University College of Physicians and Surgeons. He has collaborated with others on nearly 40 research projects dealing with the treatment of respiratory diseases.

Dr. Thomas Cate, Associate Professor of Microbiology and Immunology and of Medicine at Baylor College of Medicine in Houston, Texas, is a research physician who specializes in respiratory virus infections and the body's defenses against them.

For information about anyTime-Life book, please write:
Reader Information, Time-Life Books,
541 North Fairbanks Court, Chicago, Illinois 60611.

First printing.
Published simultaneously in Canada.
School and library distribution by Silver Burdett Company, Morristown, New Jersey.

TIME-LIFE is a trademark of Time Incorporated U.S.A.

Library of Congress Cataloguing in Publication Data
Murphy, Wendy B., 1935-
    Coping with the common cold
    (Library of Health)
    Bibliography: p.
    Includes index.
    1. Cold (Disease)    2. Influenza.
    I. Time-Life Books.    II. Title.    III. Series.
RF361.M8    616.2'05    81-1955
ISBN 0-8094-3760-0        AACR2
ISBN 0-8094-3759-7 (lib. bdg.)
ISBN 0-8094-3758-9 (ret. ed.)

Time-Life Books Inc. is a wholly owned subsidiary of
**TIME INCORPORATED**

FOUNDER: Henry R. Luce 1898-1967

Editor-in-Chief: Henry Anatole Grunwald
President: J. Richard Munro
Chairman of the Board: Ralph P. Davidson
Executive Vice President: Clifford J. Grum
Chairman, Executive Committee: James R. Shepley
Editorial Director: Ralph Graves
Group Vice President, Books: Joan D. Manley
Vice Chairman: Arthur Temple

**TIME-LIFE BOOKS INC.**

MANAGING EDITOR: Jerry Korn
Executive Editor: David Maness
Assistant Managing Editors: Dale M. Brown (planning), George Constable, Thomas H. Flaherty Jr. (acting), Martin Mann, John Paul Porter
Art Director: Tom Suzuki
Chief of Research: David L. Harrison
Director of Photography: Robert G. Mason
Assistant Art Director: Arnold C. Holeywell
Assistant Chief of Research: Carolyn L. Sackett
Assistant Director of Photography: Dolores A. Littles

CHAIRMAN: John D. McSweeney
President: Carl G. Jaeger
Executive Vice Presidents: John Steven Maxwell, David J. Walsh
Vice Presidents: George Artandi (comptroller); Stephen L. Bair (legal counsel); Peter G. Barnes; Nicholas Benton (public relations); John L. Canova; Beatrice T. Dobie (personnel); Carol Flaumenhaft (consumer affairs); James L. Mercer (Europe/South Pacific); Herbert Sorkin (production); Paul R. Stewart (marketing)

**LIBRARY OF HEALTH**

Editorial Staff for *Coping with the Common Cold*
Editor: William Frankel
Designer: Albert Sherman
Chief Researcher: Phyllis K. Wise
Picture Editor: Jane Speicher Jordan
Text Editors: Bobbie Conlan, Paul N. Mathless, David Thiemann, Steven J. Forbis, Roger E. Herst, Peter Kaufman, John Newton
Staff Writers: Jean Getlein and Rita Thievon Mullin (principals), 
Researchers: Megan Helene Barnett, Janet Doughty, Melva Morgan Holloman
Assistant Designer: Cynthia T. Richardson
Editorial Assistants: Shirley Fong Ash, Nana Varee Juarbe
Special Contributors: Barbara Hicks, Michael Roberts, Winfield Swanson

EDITORIAL PRODUCTION
Production Editor: Douglas B. Graham
Operations Manager: Gennaro C. Esposito, Gordon E. Buck (assistant)
Assistant Production Editor: Feliciano Madrid
Quality Control: Robert L. Young (director), James J. Cox (assistant), Daniel J. McSweeney, Michael G. Wight (associates)
Art Coordinator: Anne B. Landry
Copy Staff: Susan B. Galloway (chief), Margery duMond, Sheirazada Hann, Celia Beattie
Picture Department: Renée DeSandies
Traffic: Jeanne Potter

Correspondents: Elisabeth Kraemer (Bonn); Margot Hapgood, Dorothy Bacon, Lesley Coleman (London); Susan Jonas, Lucy T. Voulgaris (New York); Maria Vincenza Aloisi, Josephine du Brusle (Paris); Ann Natanson (Rome). Valuable help was also given by: Janny Hovinga (Amsterdam); Mirka Gondicas (Athens); Martha Mader (Bonn); JoAnne M. Reid (Chicago); Robert Kroon (Geneva); Bing Wong (Hong Kong); Peter Hawthorne (Johannesburg); Felix Abisheganaden (Kuala Lumpur); Judy Aspinall, Jeremy Lawrence, Karin B. Pearce, Millicent Trowbridge (London); Carolyn T. Chubet, Miriam Hsia, Christina Lieberman (New York); Mimi Murphy (Rome); Mary Johnson (Stockholm).

# CONTENTS

# CHAPTER 1

# Nothing to sneeze at

**Making sure a cold is only a cold**
**Who catches colds and when**
**First line of defense: the nose**
**A variety of viruses, all hostile**
**How the infection takes hold**

Throat sore? Head feel stuffy and dull? Nose running like a leaky faucet and you feel a chill down to your toes? No need to ask a doctor what you have, because you know only too well. You are starting another cold, maybe your second or third this year, and one of scores you have suffered and will suffer throughout your life. If you are like most people, you may wonder from time to time why, in an age of medical miracles, someone has not come up with a cure for this most persistent and most common of human afflictions. It is a sneezing, snuffling, crying shame.

Frustrated and miserable as you may feel, you can take heart in some good news about colds and other, more serious infections that resemble colds in one way or another, such as influenza *(Chapter 4)*. After centuries of folkloric humbug and decades of scientific wanderings, researchers have in recent years begun to make major discoveries about the causes of colds.

Colds, it turns out, are not a single disease that strikes over and over again but are instead perhaps as many as 200 separate, look-alike diseases, which are set in motion by any of 200 different submicroscopic agents called viruses. Cold specialists also now know a great deal about how infections are transmitted: For example, you do, indeed, ''catch'' a major share of the colds you suffer — with your hands. By touching droplets of virus-laden mucus — either on the body of a carrier who already has a cold, or on some surface that he has recently contaminated, perhaps with a sneeze or his hand — and then rubbing your own nose or eyes, you conve-

niently deliver the cold virus to the site where colds begin.

Surprisingly, colds disrupt life in tropical climates with almost the same frequency that they do in the shivery dank of temperate countries such as the United States and Great Britain; colds are rarest in those parts of the world with the lowest temperatures. So far as careful experiment can discover, there is also little direct relationship between getting wet and chilled and catching a cold. But new understanding of the body's defense mechanisms is revealing why colds, once caught, are no more than a nuisance to most people most of the time, but the first step toward serious illnesses in others.

The growing body of knowledge about viruses and their interactions with your body may eventually lead to ways of preventing and curing colds, as this knowledge already has produced treatments for influenza and many serious complications of colds. But for the moment, the central fact of ordinary colds is that no miracle cure, no antibiotic drug, no magic potion and no omniscient physician can alter the course of a cold once you have it.

Even the National Aeronautics and Space Administration has had its nose rubbed — so to speak — in this immutable fact: It can put a man into outer space, but it cannot cure the common cold. On February 27, 1969, on the eve of a flight to orbit the earth, the clockwork countdown procedure at Cape Kennedy came to an abrupt halt when all three of the Apollo 9 crew showed the classic symptoms: stuffed-up noses, sore throats and cold-related fatigue. NASA postponed the launch at an estimated cost of $500,000 — the first time in 19

*A cold sufferer blows a grotesque nose, already red, swollen and sore, in an early-19th Century French lithograph. Artists of the period frequently depicted the miseries of the ailment—sometimes with compassion, but often with harsh or flippant satire.*

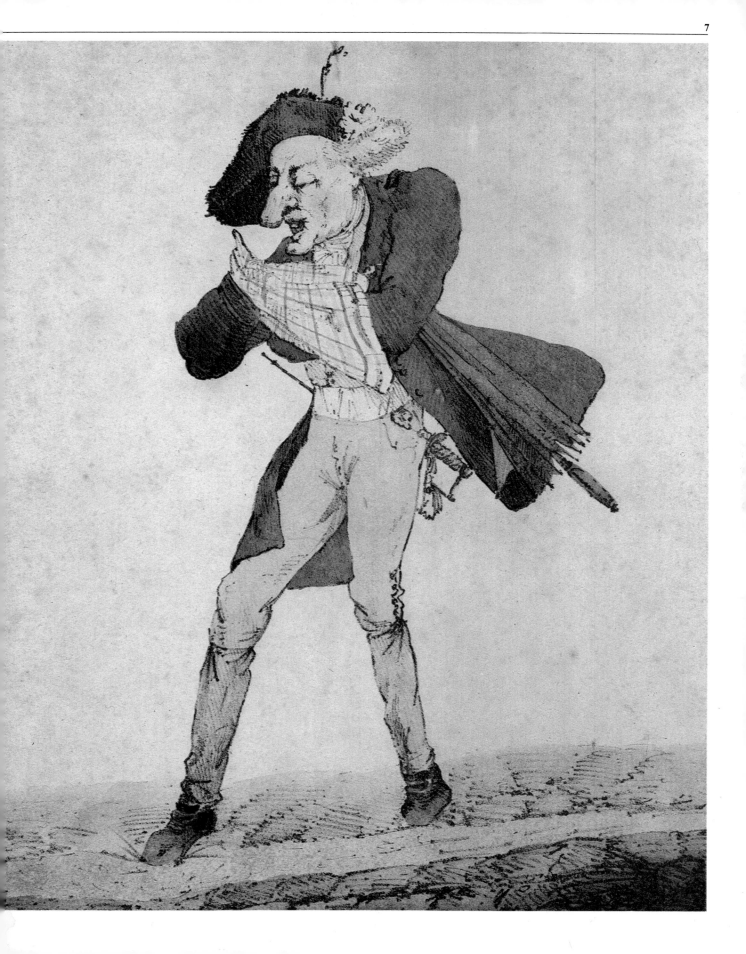

manned flights that astronaut illness, rather than bad weather or technical trouble, caused a lift-off to be delayed. The three men recovered enough to lift off on Monday, March 3 — thus confirming the adage, Treat a cold and it will end in seven days, do nothing and it will last a week. (Partly because other space crews were isolated from contamination before launch, none suffered a repetition of the expensive 1969 outbreak of the common cold.)

Apollo 9's colds may well have been the most expensive in history, but the common cold must be ranked as a costly disease in its own right. The colds contracted by Americans alone result in an estimated 300 million days of lowered efficiency, 60 million days of lost school attendance and almost 50 million days lost on the job. Add to that the money spent on cold pills, cough syrups, nose drops, visits to the doctor and mountains of tissues, and colds cost Americans about five billion dollars a year. Not surprisingly, the British and the Dutch suffer comparable losses to the affliction. Influenza, of course, can be not only costly, but deadly; in 1918 and 1919 it caused a pandemic that spread far more rapidly than the Black Death of the Middle Ages.

### Making sure a cold is only a cold

Fortunately for the world economy and the sniffling legions, most colds and influenza can be identified and treated adequately at home. The first step is to be sure that what seems to be a cold is, in fact, that transient disease and not something worse. Part of the confusion surrounding the recognition and treatment of colds stems from the multitude of words used to describe the affliction.

Physicians define a cold as an acute (fast-developing) viral infection characterized by nasal congestion (stuffiness), edema (swelling) and discharge (runny nose), and by throat irritation (sore throat). Typically, the infection is localized in the upper respiratory system, the portion of the breathing apparatus that stretches from the nostrils back and down into the upper throat (pharynx) and the voice box (larynx). Except in children, a fever is rare, and the disease is self-limiting — it takes care of itself without the intervention of doctors or medications, usually, as in the case of the Apollo 9 crew, in

about a week. But this definition, itself complex enough, is often further obfuscated by physicians and cold sufferers alike, who christen the disease exhibiting these symptoms with a number of names other than "cold."

Physicians diagnosing a cold that exhibits pronounced symptoms of runny nose and stuffiness will often call it acute coryza, from the Greek *koryza,* meaning "nasal mucus." If they have a flair for the romantic, they may also call it catarrh — from the Greek *katarrhein,* literally, "to flow down" — a holdover from the ancient belief that the nasal fluids produced during colds were secretions of a brain over-

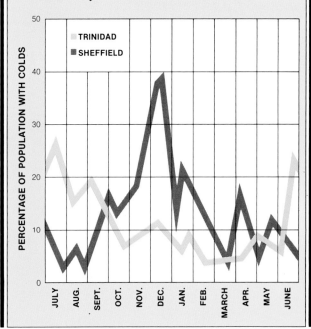

## Colds in every climate

Not surprisingly, in the Northern Hemisphere, colds reach their peak in winter: The black line in the graph below plots the prevalence of colds in Sheffield, England, during the 1960s. In the tropics colds occur most frequently during the rainy season. The Caribbean island of Trinidad *(green line),* for example, has no winter, and colds are at their worst there in June and July.

TRINIDAD
SHEFFIELD

PERCENTAGE OF POPULATION WITH COLDS

JULY AUG. SEPT. OCT. NOV. DEC. JAN. FEB. MARCH APR. MAY JUNE

burdened with waste matter. Doctors will also occasionally describe an ailment by attaching a suffix — in the case of cold symptoms, ''-itis,'' meaning inflammation — to the word for the anatomical site of the problem. Thus: rhinitis, for inflammation of the nose; pharyngitis, of the pharynx; laryngitis, of the larynx; and sinusitis, of any of the sinuses, the cavities in the bones of the skull.

Laymen use yet another set of words to describe their discomfort. A particularly confusing and popular name for a very bad cold is ''flu.'' Flu, or influenza, is indeed a severe respiratory infection, and it has many characteristics in common with a cold. But influenza is caused by a very specific group of viruses, and its impact is usually much more severe than that of a cold. Moreover, influenza is associated with widespread epidemics. Two other misleading and imprecise popular phrases are ''head cold'' and ''chest cold,'' which are supposed to distinguish a cold without a cough from a cold with a cough. A simple cold with or without a cough is essentially located in the upper respiratory tract, not in the chest; infections that involve the chest and lungs are different and more dangerous.

Just as it is not helpful to describe a bad cold as flu, neither is it wise to assume all cold symptoms are simple colds. At the least, there are imitation colds—chronic or allergic irritations of the nose and throat that persist despite the absence of infection. Many of them can be diminished or banished with medical help. More important, a great many disabling diseases start with cold symptoms. A sore throat, for example, could be a symptom of infectious mononucleosis (which can keep a patient bedridden for many weeks and leave vital organs permanently impaired) or of possibly fatal streptococcal infection.

All these ailments — whether they are secondary infections following a cold or totally unrelated diseases that only mimic a cold — are potentially far more serious than a simple cold, and they carry the risk of permanent damage to the organs involved. Many, unlike colds, can be cured or prevented with antibiotics or vaccines; in one of the frustrating paradoxes of modern medicine, the potent germ killers now available — penicillin, erythromycin and many others — can knock out infections such as strep throat and pneumonia, and polio and measles vaccines protect against those ills, but none has any effect at all on colds.

## Who catches colds and when

The symptoms of a true cold are the same for everyone, young and old, male and female, in all parts of the world. But not everyone is equally likely to suffer from them. The frequency of colds, it appears, has as much to do with who you are and what you do as with the viruses that cause the disease.

Among the social, economic and psychological factors that may play a part in susceptibility to colds, age is one of the most critical. A six-year study in Tecumseh, Michigan, made by epidemiologists at the University of Michigan School of Public Health, revealed some particulars that seem to hold true for the general population. Infants are the most cold-ridden group, averaging more than six colds and similar respiratory illnesses in the first 12 months of life. Boys have more colds than girls up to the age of three, a fact consistent with the higher rate of all illnesses among male children in those years. Preschool children who have older brothers or sisters or are themselves in day care or nursery school also get colds slightly more often than those who remain at home, where their parents are their chief contact with the outside world. After the age of three, girls are more susceptible than boys; teen-age girls average three colds a year to boys' two, and the greater susceptibility of females prevails thereafter.

The general incidence of colds continues to decline into maturity, elderly people in otherwise good health having as few as one or two colds annually. One significant exception in that declining pattern is found among people in their twenties, especially women, who show a noticeable rise in cold infections for a few years. People in this age group are most likely to have young children, and it is the youngsters who inadvertently wage germ warfare upon their parents. Adults who delay having children until their thirties and forties thereupon experience the same sudden increase in cold infections as do those who become parents in their twenties.

The Tecumseh study also found that economics plays an important role. As income increases, the frequency with

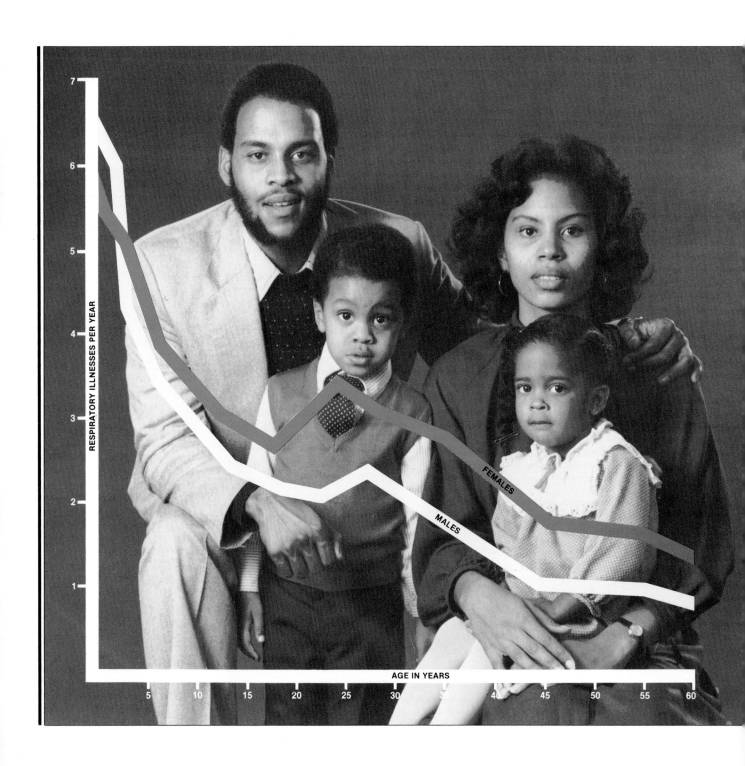

## Most susceptible: babies and women

As people grow older, they generally have fewer colds. The graph at left documents the drop-off in the incidence of respiratory disease over the average lifetime, as traced in a six-year study of 4,905 males and females in Tecumseh, Michigan. The researchers' figures lump together all respiratory illness, including influenza, bronchitis and pneumonia, as well as colds, but colds were by far the most frequent complaint.

The decline in the number of colds is not steady; a dramatic reduction in an individual's susceptibility to respiratory ailments occurs during the first 20 years of life. An average infant has a sniffly existence, suffering 6.1 colds and other respiratory infections before the age of one. By the late teens, a person will encounter only 2.5 such illnesses yearly; presumably, resistance has been stiffened by the colds endured at a younger age.

From young adulthood on, the decline in the number of annual colds continues more slowly. Respiratory ailments make a brief comeback among people in their twenties. During those child-rearing years, a couple's children are likely to pass some of their numerous colds on to the parents.

Gender makes a surprising difference. Mothers usually have closer contact with their children than fathers do, and this fact may help explain why women in their twenties and thirties experience so many more respiratory diseases than men of the same age. But elderly women and young girls are also stricken more often than males of the same ages; the only exception to this rule is boys aged three or younger. The male-female discrepancy is one of the mysteries of the common cold that continue to puzzle medical researchers.

which colds are reported within a family decreases. Families with the lowest incomes suffer about a third more colds than families at the other end of the scale. Lower income generally forces people to live in more cramped quarters than those typically occupied by wealthier people, and crowding greatly increases the opportunities for cold viruses to travel from person to person. Low income may also adversely influence diet. The degree to which poor nutrition affects susceptibility to colds is not yet clearly established, but an inadequate diet is suspected of lowering resistance generally.

There is one strange exception to the relationship between income and colds. The group that said it suffered the greatest number of respiratory illnesses is made up of families with low incomes but high levels of education. Researchers associate this surprising twist with an observation they have made over the years: Minor illnesses are largely what people make of them, and the recognition of a cold — particularly a mild one — is often a matter of self-awareness. Well-educated people are more likely to take note of and to complain about a cold than are the less educated, who tend to accept aches and pains as normal and inevitable. In fact, both low-income groups very probably have similar rates of infections.

Life style may be another critical factor in cold susceptibility. Extensive though still controversial research has suggested that people who experience great stress in their work and personal lives — who live each day on borrowed energy — can set off a chain of physiological events that inhibit the body's natural defenses against disease.

The influence of stress may account for the fact that among the subjects of the Tecumseh study, Monday, famous for being the bluest day of the week, is also the day on which most people come down with a cold. It would be easy to assume that a reluctance to go back to the job or school after the weekend is the agent of susceptibility here, but researchers believe there is another reason at work. The weekend provides a two-day incubation period during which infections contracted during the previous week can blossom into the debilitating symptoms of a cold. Thus the cold that appears full-blown on Sunday or Monday was probably contracted Thursday or Friday, when the accumulated stresses of a week's work had reduced the body's resistance to infection.

Stress may also incline some people to drink or smoke excessively, or to take sleeping pills and other drugs. Any of these can slow down, even paralyze, defensive reflexes that normally protect the upper respiratory tract. For the same reason, chemical pollutants in the air also may make people more susceptible to upper respiratory infections. In some instances, pollutants may inhibit the body's defense mechanisms or irritate the nasal membranes that ordinarily protect against infection. In other cases, pollutants can initiate an allergic reaction, causing symptoms that mimic those of a cold but are not caused by a cold virus.

The role played by air quality in cold infections is relatively simple compared with broader effects of the environment. Researchers have tried all sorts of diabolical schemes for testing the widely held belief that certain climates and weather conditions make people more likely to catch cold — and as far as they have been able to discover, there is no direct relationship. In one study undertaken at the Common Cold Unit, a British center that began studying the disease in 1946, volunteers were divided into three groups. One group was inoculated with an infectious solution of cold viruses and then required to stand around in a cold room in dripping-wet bathing suits for a half hour. A second group was not administered the virus solution but did get the same miserable treatment with cold rooms and soggy suits. The last group was inoculated like the first but otherwise left alone. Group 2 — chilled but not inoculated — developed no colds within the usual incubation period. The inoculated groups — chilled and unchilled alike — did succumb and at about the same rate.

Similar results were obtained by American cold researchers Drs. H. F. Dowling and George Gee Jackson among groups of shivering Chicagoans in 1957, with one interesting exception: Women in the middle third of their menstrual cycle were found to be dramatically more susceptible to colds following chilling. About 77 per cent of them developed colds when inoculated with cold viruses and exposed to chilling conditions as compared with only 29 per cent of the other women. Dowling and Jackson believed this to show that

hormonal changes in the susceptible group had produced significant — though as yet unidentifiable — changes in the mucous membranes of the nose.

Perhaps even more difficult to sort out is the so-called winter factor in susceptibility to colds. Colds and cold weather are widely believed to be related; presumably that ancient notion is the basis for calling such diseases colds in the first place. But low temperatures are now known to play a relatively minor role; what matters is the season.

One study found that the annual rate of cold and other respiratory infections for students in the semitropical Philippines was more than twice as high as that for students in Wisconsin, where winters are long and bitter: 49 per 1,000 compared with 24 per 1,000. But the study also found that in both places the peak of infections occurred during the cooler part of the year — the rainy season in the Philippines, fall and winter in Wisconsin.

The mysterious winter factor thus seems to be at work, but there is no unshakable theory yet as to precisely how it works. Many researchers ascribe the connection to a change in behavior patterns. In both temperate and tropical climates, the season of inclement weather coincides with the return to school and an increase in the hours spent indoors — where crowded quarters and poor air circulation would make it easier to pass on infection.

Other research shows that within the colder months in places like North America, there are three peak periods of cold infection — coinciding roughly with the arrival of seasonal changes in fall, midwinter and spring. Some scientists think these turns in the weather may create just enough physiological stress to upset the body's ability to keep cold viruses in check. Others blame psychological stresses, noting that one of the three peaks in cold infections in Western Europe and the United States occurs at the Christmas-New Year's holiday season, a time that is supposed to be pleasant but actually is one of intense emotional stress.

That the winter factor has little to do with external air temperature is indicated by the experience of people who live in areas of extreme cold. One of the most infection-free places on the globe is the South Pole, where temperatures fall

# A rapid-transit route for the breath of life

The cold-prone human respiratory tract, simplified in drawings at right and on the following pages, is about 16 inches long in the average adult, made up of bones, muscles and cartilage and packed with glands, tubes, folds and flaps. Yet inhaled air takes less than two thirds of a second to travel the entire route.

The journey starts in an antechamber, the nose, where the air swirls for a quarter second or so. Special cells in the nasal cavity provide the sense of smell; tiny openings link the cavity to air-filled spaces in the skull called sinuses *(page 18)*. Other openings link the nose to the eyes through the nasolacrimal ducts *(page 41)*, and to the ears through the Eustachian tubes *(page 83)*.

From the nose, in a leg of its trip that lasts less than $^1/_{10}$ second, air flows swiftly through the pharynx, or throat, and down into the larynx, or voice box. In the larynx a set of vibrating flaps, the vocal cords, turns a rush of air into sound, and a valve prevents food and liquid from entering the airway.

The last stage of the trip is the slowest—a third of a second. The air goes down the trachea (windpipe) to tubes called bronchi and fans out into the lungs. There the breath—warmed or cooled, moistened, and cleansed of particles carrying bacteria and viruses—fulfills the purpose of the entire system: The air gives up oxygen to feed the body, and takes on carbon dioxide for the return trip.

**A MAP OF THE AIRWAYS**
*The linked airways of the respiratory tract begin at the nose and mouth. Beyond lies the pharynx, studded with clumps of protective tissue called tonsils and adenoids (page 19). At the larynx food is diverted to the stomach and air is directed through the trachea to the bronchi, which branch off into the lungs.*

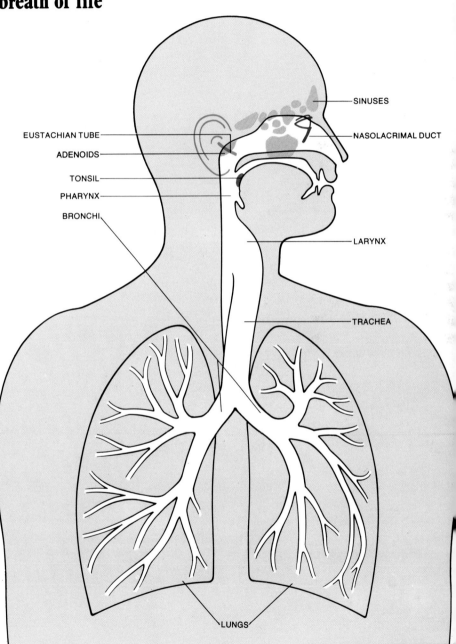

EUSTACHIAN TUBE
ADENOIDS
TONSIL
PHARYNX
BRONCHI
SINUSES
NASOLACRIMAL DUCT
LARYNX
TRACHEA
LUNGS

14

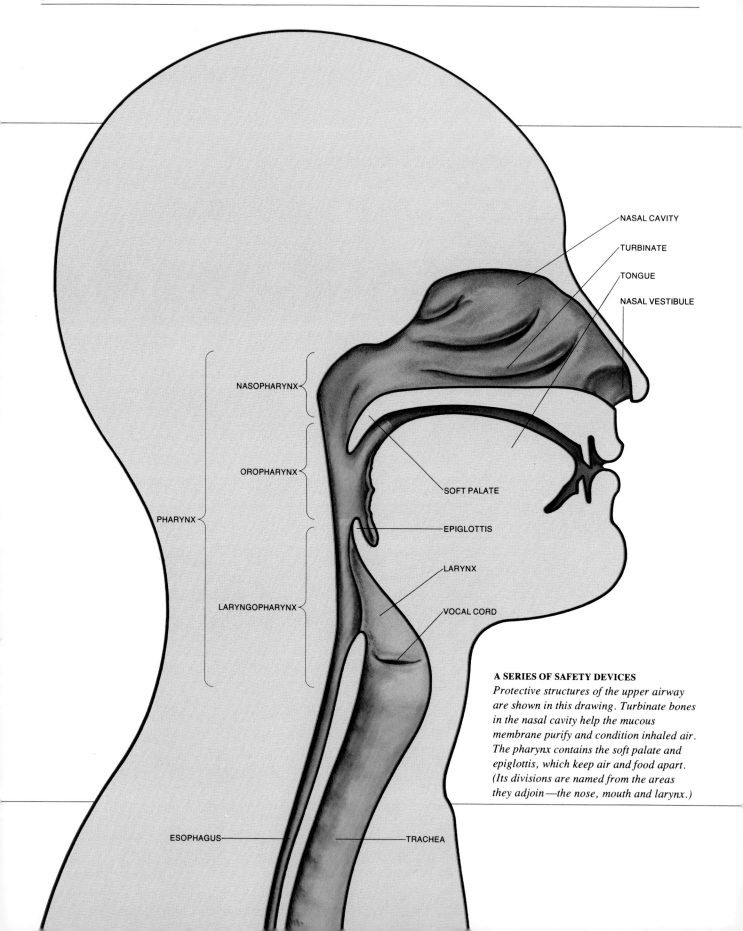

NASAL CAVITY

TURBINATE

TONGUE

NASAL VESTIBULE

NASOPHARYNX

OROPHARYNX

SOFT PALATE

PHARYNX

EPIGLOTTIS

LARYNX

VOCAL CORD

LARYNGOPHARYNX

**A SERIES OF SAFETY DEVICES**
*Protective structures of the upper airway
are shown in this drawing. Turbinate bones
in the nasal cavity help the mucous
membrane purify and condition inhaled air.
The pharynx contains the soft palate and
epiglottis, which keep air and food apart.
(Its divisions are named from the areas
they adjoin—the nose, mouth and larynx.)*

ESOPHAGUS

TRACHEA

# Safeguards of the upper airway

Every day an average adult breathes in and out about 22,000 times, inhaling and exhaling some 500 cubic feet of air. Along with essential oxygen come dirt, pollen and disease germs—and, over part of the breathing route, food. The upper airway *(opposite),* which conducts this enormous volume of air from the nose to the windpipe, is designed to remove, divert or neutralize these contaminants and simultaneously adjust air temperature and humidity to internal requirements.

The nose provides the first line of defense against airborne threats. Short, thick hairs just inside the nostrils filter out the larger particles. Most of the smaller particles are trapped—stuck like flies on flypaper—by the mucous membrane, which lines the nasal cavity and most of the airway down into the lungs. This protective lining, the part of the system most affected by a cold, is covered with invisibly small hairs, or cilia—as many as 250 to one membrane cell. They are continuously blanketed by mucus, the viscous secretion of the glands within the membrane.

Inside the nose, the area that incoming air must pass over is increased by projections called turbinates, scroll-like bones sticking into the passageway from the side. They not only present more mucus for more effective trapping of dirt but also increase the contact between the air and the membrane's network of blood vessels, which warm or cool the air.

Incoming air reaching the pharynx must be separated from food, which also moves through this part of the passageway. This tricky operation often goes awry, producing fits of coughing when food goes down the wrong way. Protecting the airway from food is the job of the epiglottis, a one-way valve that moves during a swallow to close off the larynx and shunt food into the esophagus, on its way to the stomach below.

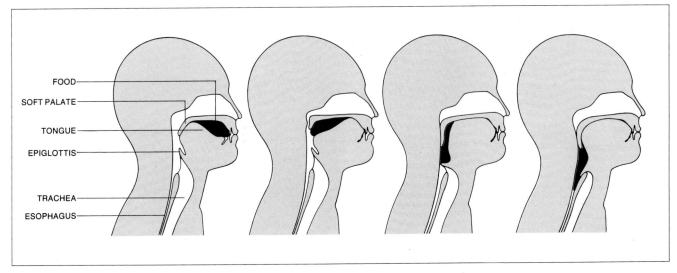

FOOD
SOFT PALATE
TONGUE
EPIGLOTTIS
TRACHEA
ESOPHAGUS

**THE MECHANISM OF A SWALLOW**
*These four drawings, depicting the stages of a single swallow from beginning to end, indicate how food is kept out of the airway of the respiratory tract. In the first drawing, food is taken into the mouth; in the second, the tongue pushes the food back toward the throat, and a reflex action tilts the soft palate to seal off the opening between the mouth and the nose. Then the leaf-shaped epiglottis valve folds down over the entrance to the larynx, blocking the passage to the lungs (third drawing). Breathing ceases for a moment and, as shown in the fourth drawing, the food is moved down into the esophagus.*

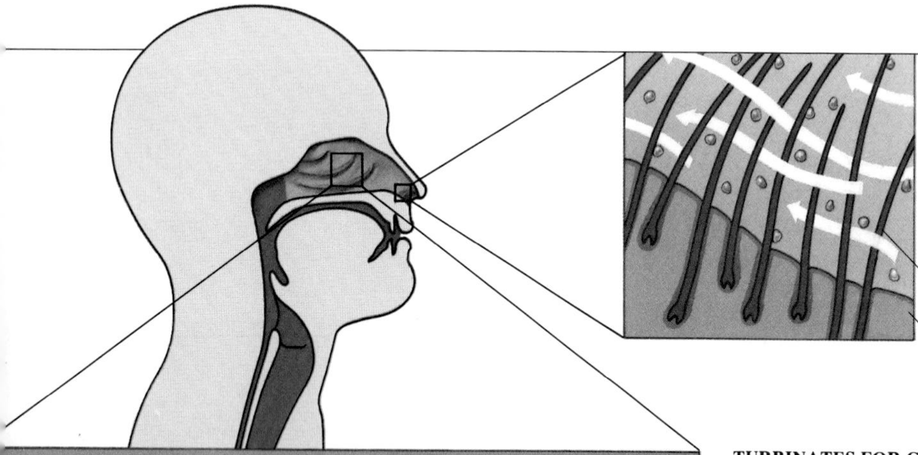

## HAIR FOR COARSE CLEANING

*As air is inhaled (arrows), stiff hairs called vibrissae, growing from the nasal lining at the entrance to the nose, trap the larger particles carried in the airstream. These nasal hairs filter out most of the dust, dirt and grit that enter the nose.*

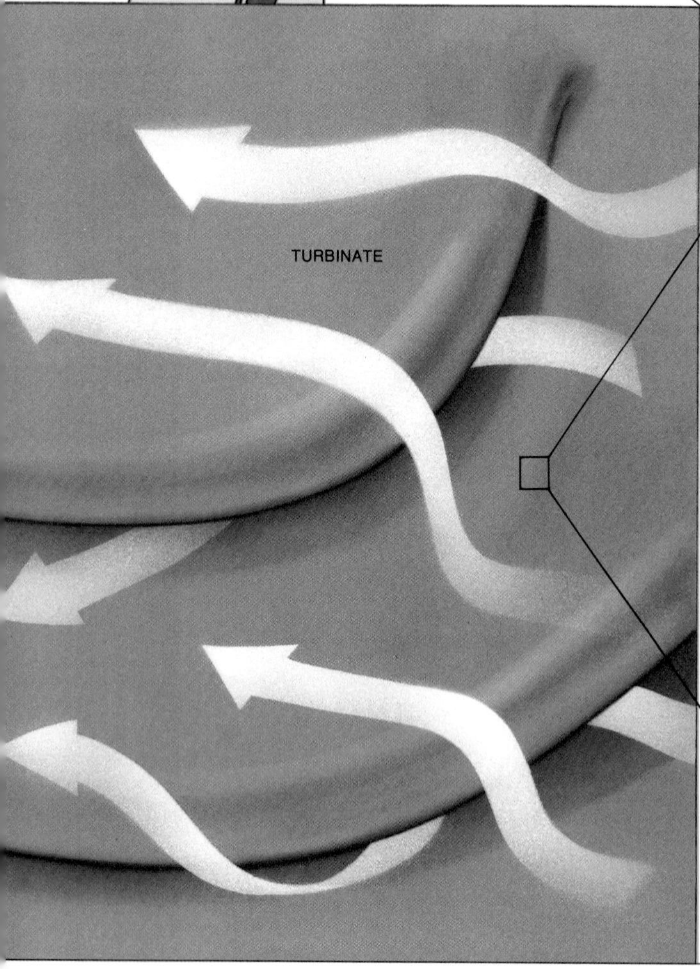

NASAL HAIR
NASAL LINING

## TURBINATES FOR CONDITIONING

*Inhaled air (arrows) passes between the bony structures called turbinates, which project from the side walls of the nose. In a split second, blood vessels in the mucous membrane covering the turbinates warm the air almost to body temperature, and mucus moistens it to 75 to 80 per cent relative humidity.*

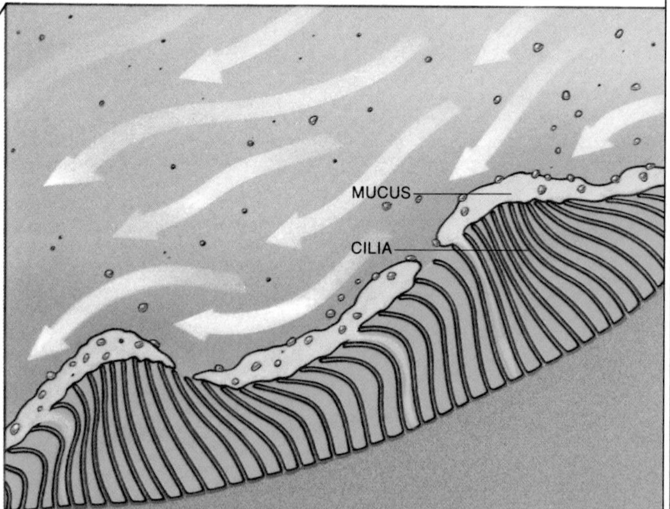

TURBINATE

MUCUS
CILIA
MUCOUS MEMBRANE

## MUCUS FOR FINE CLEANING AND PURIFYING

*Patches of sticky mucus entrap particles too small to be caught by the nasal hairs. At the same time, cilia—tiny lashing filaments growing from the mucous membrane—propel the mucus to the throat at about a quarter inch a minute. The mucus is swallowed, and its contents are destroyed in the stomach.*

to -100° F. Colds were found to be a rarity among the scientists who maintain a research station there. When colds did occur, they could usually be directly traced to the arrival of a newcomer or the return of someone who had been home on leave. And once one person at the station succumbed, virtually everyone else did, too, in quick order. The scientists' isolation, a kind of inadvertent quarantine, may be the controlling factor in this pattern of infection, in which long periods relatively free of illness result in a lowered immunity to viral infection — which in turn leads to an outbreak of colds when a virus is introduced from the outside. This pattern, once typical in all seasonally inaccessible places, whatever their climates, is becoming less common as transportation to all corners of the earth improves.

**First line of defense: the nose**

Although scientists isolated at the South Pole may not catch colds often, when they do they get the disease the same way as a three-year-old who always seems to have a runny nose: A virus enters any of the passages leading to the throat and infects the tissues there. The most important of these passages is the nose. It is the first point of contact between harmful airborne substances and the body's defenses against them. Its primary functions are to warm, moisturize and filter the roughly 500 cubic feet of air breathed each day — the equivalent of all the air contained in an empty room measuring 6 by 10 by 8 feet. The nose also acts as a resonance chamber for the voice. Finally—and almost incidentally in the human species—the nose functions as the organ of smell.

To carry out all these jobs successfully in so small an area requires that the architecture of the nose be extremely complex and efficient. The interior of the nose is divided into two chambers by a partition called the septum, made up of bone and a more flexible material called cartilage. With the possible exception of the Greek goddess Aphrodite, virtually no one has a perfectly shaped septum that divides the nose beautifully down the middle. In most mortals, the septum deviates to one side or the other, making one chamber slightly smaller — and slightly more prone to congestion — than the other.

Protruding partway from the outer walls of each chamber are three curled ridges or plates of bone that further subdivide the nasal cavity. Called turbinates, these plates multiply the nose's interior wall surfaces many times over. The surfaces are lined with a multilayered mucous membrane, which actually performs most of the nose's duties as resident air conditioner. This membrane is crammed with small blood vessels. Inhaled air passing over and around the turbinates is thus exposed to volumes of circulating blood and even in 10° F. weather is warmed to about 91° before it reaches the top of the throat. In very hot weather, the blood vessels help absorb heat from the torrid air so that the air is cooled and does not damage the lungs. The top layer of mucous-membrane cells, along with glands embedded in the membrane, carry out the nose's humidifying — and, when necessary, cooling — action by constantly secreting a sticky fluid called mucus (hence the adjective "mucous"), more than a pint of it a day. The mucus may contribute about a pint of water per day to inhaled air, maintaining a relative humidity in the nose as high as 80 per cent.

This blanket of mucus is an essential protection against colds. It acts as a buffer between the upper respiratory system and irritating substances that may enter along with inhaled air. The mucus defends the tissue beneath it from a range of invaders — everything from dust particles to germs — either by destroying them with enzymes and other body chemicals or by keeping them suspended away from the vulnerable cells of the membrane until they are swallowed. An army of minute, hairlike cilia (not to be confused with the coarse visible hairs that screen the front of the nostrils against large airborne particles) continually advances the mucus through the intricate passageways of the nose. Beating as often as 1,000 times per minute, the cilia deliver the mucus blanket to the back of the mouth and eventually into the digestive tract, where it and its irritating passengers are destroyed by digestive fluids in the stomach.

Within the membrane is a small patch of nerve cells that take care of the sense of smell, transmitting their reactions to the brain along tiny nerve fibers. When you have a cold and your nose is congested and inflamed, these cells are often put out of action. Meals then seem disappointingly pallid, because what you can taste is always largely a matter of what you can smell—and with a cold you cannot smell very much.

Accessories to the marvelously efficient nasal machine are the sinuses, four groups of cavities in the bones of the skull *(below).* Two sinuses are located over the eyes, just above the eyebrows. Two others are just behind the bridge of the nose; just behind them, deep within the head, is another. The largest of the four groups lies in the cheekbones just below the eyes. These air-filled cavities serve to protect the brain from blows to the front of the head. They are lined with mucous membrane, which serves as a supplemental source of mucus if for some reason the nasal secretions are inadequate. The sinuses normally drain into the nasal cavity through narrow canals. However, a cold or an allergic reaction can make the mucous membrane swell and block the canals, building up pressure that causes severe headaches.

Quite separate in function from the respiratory system but also important in colds are the tear ducts, located on either side of the bridge of the nose. They carry away the excess moisture produced by glands that constantly clean and lubricate the eyes. Like the sinuses, the tear ducts drain into the nasal cavity— which is why the seemingly innocent gesture of rubbing your eyes with your hands can give a cold virus entry into your body.

Behind and below the nasal cavity is the part of the throat called the pharynx, a vertical, nearly round passageway about five inches long in adults. The pharynx shuttles air toward the lungs while sending food, mucus and other materials toward the stomach.

The pharynx is also lined with mucous membrane to continue the work of warming, moisturizing and cleansing the air in the upper respiratory system. By the time air reaches the lungs, it will be close to normal body temperature and almost saturated with water.

Within the pharynx are two distinctly separate masses of spongy tissue, the tonsils and adenoids *(opposite),* which can be infected by viruses or bacteria. The tonsils, small, reddish, oval-shaped structures, lie at the base of the tongue, just behind the last lower molars. The adenoids, somewhat larger, are stationed on the roof of the throat at the back of the nasal passageways. Both the tonsils and the adenoids grow to their maximum size in early childhood. If left alone, they generally shrink after puberty until they all but disappear in adulthood.

Long regarded as unnecessary relics of evolution— and major sources of spreading infection— they were in past times routinely removed when a child reached his fourth or fifth year. Now, however, physicians usually leave these glands in place unless they become abnormally enlarged and repeatedly inflamed. Far from being useless appendages, the tonsils and adenoids actually are islands of defense, part of the body's system for combating disease. They store the white blood cells that attack and remove any foreign invaders, and they also release specific agents designed to defend the body against certain viruses and bacteria.

Close by the adenoids are the two Eustachian tubes, which lead from the middle chamber of each ear into the upper throat. The tubes are air passages, designed to keep the pressure on the outside of the eardrum equal to that within the semi-enclosed middle ear. During a cold, infection can spread up into the Eustachian tubes and cause earaches.

And at the lower end of the upper respiratory system, just below the pharynx, is the larynx, or voice box, a valve that controls the passage of air. A pair of cordlike ligaments stretching across this valve vibrate to create the voice. Mu-

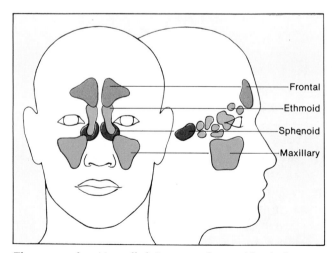

*The groups of cavities called sinuses, each named for the bone in which it appears, are anatomical mysteries — some scientists believe they are voice resonators, others that they lighten the skull. Their potential for trouble, however, is well understood: Membranes swollen by a cold may block sinus drainage passages, making the cavities incubators of bacterial infection.*

cous membrane extends from the nose and pharynx over the larynx walls. Inflammation of this membrane produces the hoarseness or loss of voice that accompanies some colds.

## A variety of viruses, all hostile

Enter the viruses, to disrupt all the normally smooth-running parts of the upper respiratory system. As compared with bacteria, the other main category of disease germs that trouble humanity, viruses are markedly smaller and simpler. A typical bacterium — a streptococcus, for example — is too small to be seen with the naked eye but is easily visible under a conventional schoolroom microscope. Most viruses, by contrast — including those that cause colds — are about a hundred times smaller, perhaps a ten-millionth of an inch across, and are clearly visible only under the extreme magnification of an electron microscope.

In terms of complexity, a bacterium is a complete, living organism, a single-celled member of the plant kingdom, while a virus is so simple in structure as to make even its classification as a living body debatable. Under the microscope, a virus resembles a snowflake or a mineral crystal, for its shape is geometrically regular, like a many-sided box or a spiral. Unlike a bacterium, a virus has no mechanism for movement, no internal method of reproduction, no equipment for ingesting or digesting food — in short, none of the

abilities generally considered minimum requirements for membership in the world of the living. A virus cannot even qualify as a cell. It is rather an assemblage of various chemicals that enable more new structures exactly like the virus to be produced, all surrounded by a protective protein shell.

A virus cannot even cause such duplication on its own. Only when the virus gets into living tissue can it multiply. Then it takes over its host, using the living cell's own substance to produce more virus particles. The virus is very fussy about its unwilling host; for each kind of virus there is only one general kind of cell that the virus can subject to its rule. Its protein shell can form attachments to receptors on the surfaces of only one particular kind of host cell — rather like a key that will turn only in the lock designed for it.

This so-called specificity determines the seriousness of the disease induced by a given virus. The rabies virus, for example, becomes a considerable threat to life because it takes hold in brain tissue. The polio virus sometimes lodges in the spinal cord and brain stem. Still other viruses selectively infect skin, glands or gastrointestinal tract, causing warts, mumps or a form of diarrhea. Cold viruses, on the other hand, are keyed to attach themselves to the cells of the mucous membrane of the respiratory tract. The viruses destroy these cells one by one, but because the cells are located in tissue that is itself relatively superficial, the loss of these cells brings discomfort but seldom anything worse.

The cells of the upper respiratory tract can be attacked by some 200 different cold viruses. Identifying the one causing a particular cold is a painstaking, expensive process, and the technique involved is not readily available to the average doctor. Nor would it be of much use even if it were: There is no way to make a cold go away any faster by picking its perpetrator out of a viral line-up. But the ability to distinguish one cold virus from another is basic to the continuing search for methods of prevention, and the process is still unfolding.

Many of the cold viruses share several identifying characteristics in addition to their affinity for the cells of the upper respiratory system. For example, the rhino viruses, responsible for as many as half of all colds, multiply best at a temperature of 91° F., in an environment that is less acid than kitchen

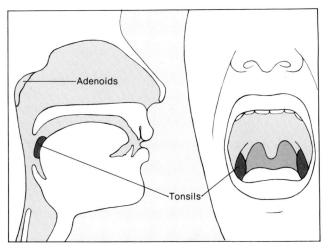

*The tonsils and adenoids are areas in which biochemical defenses called antibodies are produced to fight infection. The tonsils are a matched pair at the sides of the throat, the adenoids a single mass high at the back. Paradoxically, both may become infected and cause infection elsewhere, particularly in childhood, when tonsils and adenoids are at their largest.*

**CORONA VIRUS**
*The second largest cause of colds, corona viruses were discovered in 1965 and named for their crownlike circlets, which resemble a solar corona. They are spread in airborne droplets from coughs and sneezes, and tend to strike in midwinter.*

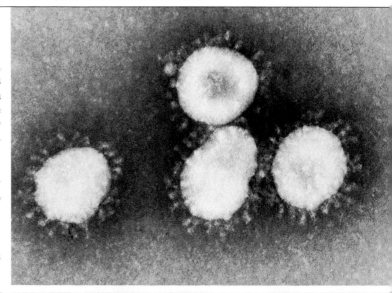

# A rogue's gallery of viruses

After years of searching for a single, elusive common-cold virus, scientists have discovered not one virus, but eight different groups including more than 200 viruses that can cause the illness called a cold—and sometimes flu or worse. All eight groups share one insidious trait: an affinity for the human respiratory tract. In every other way they vary widely, as can be seen from these photographs, in which each virus is magnified about 200,000 times.

Two viral groups, rhino virus *(below)* and corona virus *(right),* account for about half of all colds; the other six groups cause only about 10 per cent, leaving the cause of the remainder—about two out of every five colds—a mystery yet to be solved. Meanwhile, the full roles of the known cold viruses are still being explored. One discovery: Respiratory syncytial virus *(opposite, top left)* causes colds in adults, but pneumonia and bronchiolitis in infants and small children.

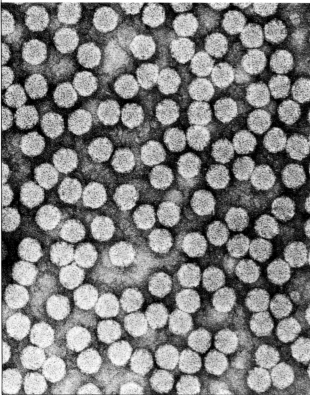

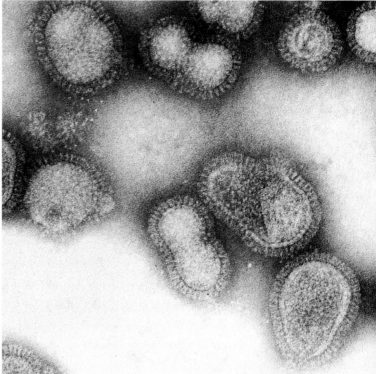

**RHINO VIRUS**
*Named from the Greek for "nose," where its effects are felt, but looking like geodesic domes, rhino viruses spread by direct contact. More than 100 types infect human hosts the year round, causing more colds than any other group of viruses.*

**INFLUENZA VIRUS**
*Three types of influenza virus, subdivided into many strains, cause colds and flu. All are round, about four billionths of an inch in diameter (medium size for a virus) and studded with spikes. Type A, the most common and dangerous, is shown above.*

**RESPIRATORY SYNCYTIAL VIRUS**
*Generally spherical and always covered with spiky projections, this cold virus strikes in winter. It produces lower respiratory tract illness in infants and small children.*

**PARAINFLUENZA VIRUS**
*Largest of cold viruses (up to 12 billionths of an inch in diameter), parainfluenza viruses cause colds that in infants and children may lead to croup or pneumonia. These particles broke open as they were prepared for viewing, and hereditary material poured out.*

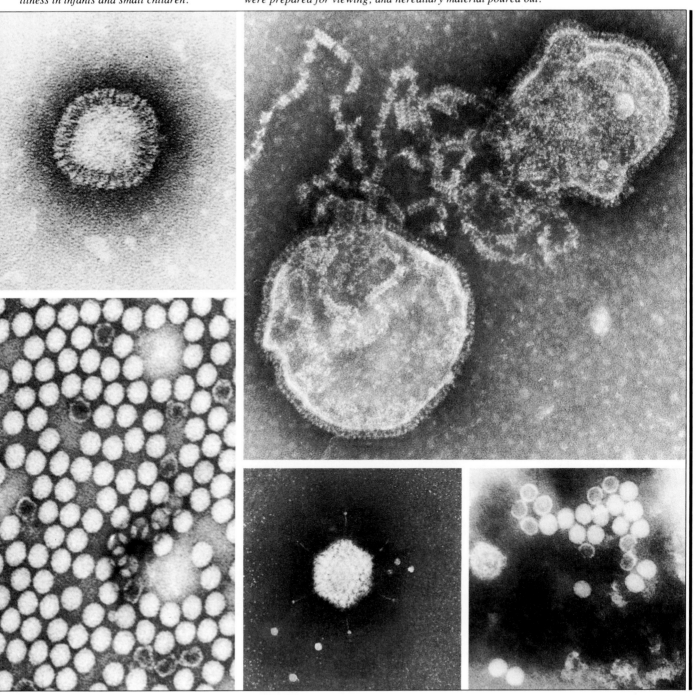

**COXSACKIE VIRUS**
*These viruses have 20 facets, invisible even at 200,000-times magnification. Named for the New York town where they were discovered, they cause colds with fever.*

**ADENO VIRUS**
*Intricate assemblages of facets and knob-tipped rods, adeno viruses produce late-winter, spring and early-summer colds, but rarely attack people over 15.*

**ECHO VIRUS**
*Close cousins of the coxsackie viruses and identical in structure, echo viruses cause colds accompanied by fever, sore throats and severe coughs, especially in children.*

vinegar, and in the presence of a rich supply of oxygen. This combination of conditions is precisely met in the nose and nowhere else in the body. But cold viruses also have certain other features that enable laboratory technicians to tell them apart, and to identify a given virus as a member of one of several groups or families that are as different in shape and size from one another as robins are from giraffes.

Most colds that can be linked to a specific virus group are caused by rhino viruses, all shaped like a gemstone cut with 20 equal facets but differing in chemical make-up—there are more than 100 distinct types. They have been found to be particularly significant as agents of late-summer colds and the annual autumn cold epidemic that coincides with the resumption of school. Two related types, coxsackie and echo, identical in size and shape, occasionally cause summer colds but are generally responsible for serious illnesses such as meningitis, pleurisy and a heart disease called pericarditis.

The next common cause of colds is made up of corona viruses, so called because they are round or elliptical and covered with projections that form a kind of corona, or crown. Corona viruses are most prevalent in winter and may spread in epidemics—often a single type is responsible for almost every cold in a particular geographic area.

Other major virus groups thus far implicated in colds include the adeno viruses, named for the fact that examples were first isolated in a child's adenoids. Viruses of this group

## Facts and fancies about catching colds

Careful scientific investigation has debunked many firmly held beliefs about the causes of colds—fatigue, wet and chill, for example, seem to have no effect. But some of grandmother's cautions have been upheld, such as the advisability of covering sneezes and coughs. Below is a selection of presumed facts, some true, some false and some still in doubt.

CHILDREN CATCH MORE COLDS THAN ANYONE ELSE.
*True.* Not only do young children suffer more colds, but parents with young children get more colds than other people their age.

KISSING IS A SURE WAY TO SPREAD A COLD.
*False.* Colds are rather difficult to catch by way of the mouth. University of Wisconsin researchers tested couples, asking that in each couple, the cold-stricken partner kiss the unafflicted one for 90 seconds. Only one caught cold.

ADULTS TEND TO GET FEWER COLDS AS THEY GROW OLDER.
*True.* The older a person is, the more likely it is that he already has had a particular cold virus and has some immunity to it.

SMOKERS CATCH MORE COLDS THAN NONSMOKERS.
*False.* Several studies have shown that both groups are equally susceptible. However, their symptoms differ. Smokers develop coughs more often than nonsmokers, and the cough persists longer; nonsmokers more often have a sore, scratchy throat.

ADULTS WHOSE TONSILS WERE REMOVED IN CHILDHOOD GET WORSE COLDS THAN THOSE WHO STILL HAVE THEIR TONSILS.
*False.* Laboratory experiments with volunteers given virus-laden nose drops showed that a tonsillectomy affected neither susceptibility to colds nor the severity of colds that were contracted.

HAY-FEVER SUFFERERS GET PARTICULARLY BAD COLDS.
*True.* Experiments on those afflicted with this allergy indicated that their colds were more severe than those of other people.

INTROVERTS SUFFER WORSE COLDS THAN OUTGOING, EXTROVERTED PERSONALITY TYPES.
*Probably true.* When volunteers at Britain's Common Cold Unit were rated with standard psychological tests, scientists found introverts did indeed get worse cold symptoms than extroverts. Introverts also spread more virus particles, another indication that their infections were more severe.

ONGOING STRESS, SUCH AS A HIGH-PRESSURE JOB, INCREASES VULNERABILITY TO COLDS.
*Probably false.* Studies at the Common Cold Unit found that sudden psychological jolts, rather than continuing stress, heightened susceptibility to colds. The true culprit seems to be the stress associated with change itself, whether the change is positive or negative; thus any major disruption of routine—even a pleasant diversion such as a vacation—increases the risk of a cold.

are relatively large, with 20 facets that take a branching, snowflake-like form. Like virtually all cold viruses, these favor particular seasons, being most active in late winter, early spring and early summer, but of negligible significance in midsummer. In adults adeno viruses produce ordinary colds at most. More than half of the infections detected in community studies were subclinical—that is, they produced no signs of sickness in the individual, and aborted quietly without so much as a handkerchief being raised. But in children, whose immune systems are not yet fully developed, the adeno viruses can cause more severe respiratory infections such as bronchitis and pneumonia. And in the closed populations of training camps, adeno viruses may also spread rapidly to lay low an entire military community.

Another three groups of viruses—all relatively large and rounded—can bring on cold symptoms varying in severity. One group includes the microorganisms responsible for influenza, which in milder forms can be indistinguishable from a common cold. The very similar parainfluenza viruses do not cause influenza but produce colds. In adults, parainfluenza is generally mild, but can be more serious for children, causing respiratory diseases ranging from croup to an inflammation of the lungs called bronchiolitis. In infants and young children, both infections are also caused by another related microorganism, the respiratory syncytial virus.

Scientists currently regard rhino viruses as agents of some 30 to 50 per cent of common colds in adults, perhaps somewhat fewer in children. Corona viruses, they believe, cause another 15 to 20 per cent, while viruses of the other families are blamed for another 10 per cent. This leaves 20 to 45 per cent of upper respiratory infections with specific causes that are still unknown. Virologists continue to look for viral villains in the hope that by learning to recognize them and their precise methods of infecting the respiratory tract they will also find clues as to how medicine might intervene.

## The perfect parasite

The process by which viruses cause colds is intricate and all the more fascinating because so much of it is, essentially, invisible. A cold virus in isolation can be seen under an electron microscope, but once it begins its work in a host cell, it disappears from view. Soon after it attaches itself to the appropriate host, this perfect parasite penetrates the cell wall. The virus then loses its protective coating and reprograms the reproductive activities of the cell. Now, instead of continuing to sustain or propagate itself, the hapless host cell begins to produce more enemy viruses. A crowded virus factory, the cell may burst open, releasing up to a thousand new and identical viruses into the surrounding tissue, and these will repeat the infectious process again and again. The exhausted host cell, its internal structure a shambles, is left, usually to die.

People repeatedly suffer such viral insults, quite often with little more than a vague sense of malaise or with no sensation at all. In these cases, the body's protective forces may have quietly and successfully marshaled to encircle the invaders before they can spread very far. Thwarted, the viruses infect fewer and fewer cells, and the "inapparent," or subclinical, infection comes to a symptom-free end.

If the body's initial reaction to the invasion was inadequate, however, thousands of viruses soon multiply into millions, leaving in their wake a trail of broken cells. One to four days after the onslaught of the infection, the misery of a cold sets in.

Charles Lamb, the 19th Century essayist, summed up the result for every human plagued by this ubiquitous disease when he described his own suffering: "Do you know what it is to succumb to an insurmountable day mare—a wholesome lethargy—an indisposition to do anything—a total deadness and distaste—a suspension of vitality—an indifference to locality—a numb soporifical goodfornothingness—an ossification all over—an oyster-like insensibility to the passing events—a mind stupor—a brawny defiance to the needles of a thrusting-in conscience? Who shall deliver me from the body of this death?"

Unfortunately for Lamb, no one in his time could suggest any effective means of deliverance. But, as reported in the following chapter, there are today a number of constructive ways to stay healthy and avoid colds, not all colds certainly, but some. ❄

# Traditional treatments: some help, some do not

Most people, in most parts of the world, treat upper respiratory infections much as their ancestors did thousands of years ago — with herbs, amulets and a variety of practices either unrelated or only tenuously related to those of modern medicine. Some of these traditional treatments (like folk treatments for other ailments) have actually shown real effectiveness in relieving the symptoms of the disease. Others are clearly useless — though they sometimes serve as innocuous or mildly painful distractions from an ailment that is, in any case, self-limiting and short-lived.

Dry cupping, shown at right, is an example of the distraction school of folk medicine. Traditional in Greece, Mexico, Vietnam and other parts of the world, dry cupping grew out of the ancient practice of bloodletting, in which a vein is cut and blood is either allowed to flow or sucked out through gourds or hollow horns (in a process called wet cupping) or by leeches; in theory, the drawn blood drains disease from the body.

By comparison, dry cupping is a mild remedy, with little risk beyond a few blisters or broken capillaries. Its theory is that cures can be effected simply by drawing blood to the skin and away from a diseased organ. Medically, its effect is that of a counterirritant. Like a mustard plaster, another favorite cold remedy, it produces such warmth and stinging on the surface of the skin that a cold is likely to be forgotten, at least temporarily.

Two other traditional therapies with distinguished lineages are shown on the following pages: herbal medicines, which are older than humankind (many animals instinctively medicate themselves with grasses and herbs), and acupuncture, a system of treatment, part metaphysical, part empirical, developed by the Chinese more than 7,000 years ago. Acupuncture has since found favor throughout Asia, and its extraordinary successes in treating a broad range of diseases have led many Westerners to investigate its somewhat mysterious processes.

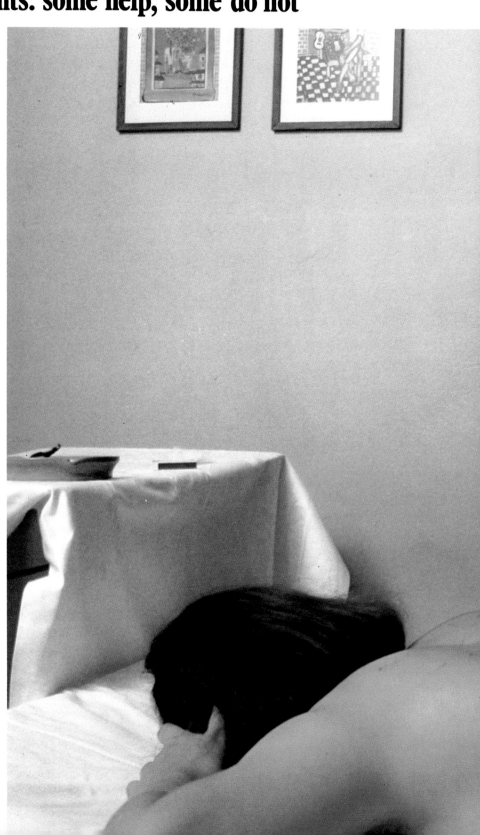

*A Greek patient with a respiratory ailment submits to dry cupping. Using traditional methods, her practitioner heats two cups and sets them on the patient's skin. Each cup raises a dome of skin as the heated air inside it cools and contracts; then the cups are removed, reheated and reset. For a cold the entire procedure takes about 15 minutes.*

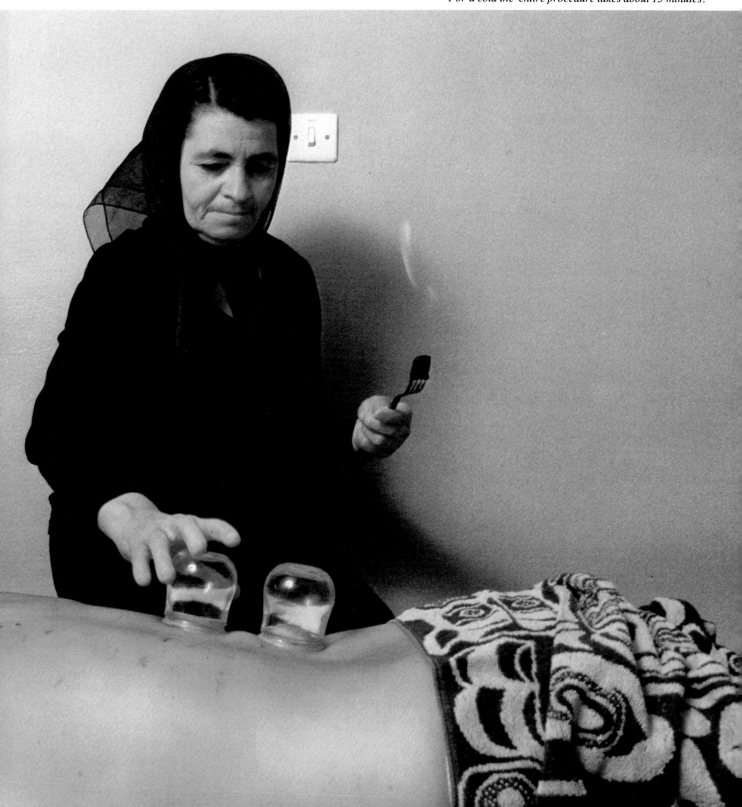

# Medicines from nature's pharmacy

Among the peoples who have used herbs to treat disease, few have had a longer or richer record of success than American Indians.

While particular herbs are the active ingredients of most Indian remedies, the treatment of each disease — even mundane colds and flu — is closely linked to tribal religious beliefs and mythology in a process that requires the arts and wisdom of a medicine man for maximum effect. When relief or a cure results, scientists using conventional Western standards of evidence sometimes find it difficult to tell whether the improvement is mainly physical or psychological.

Dramatic examples of Indian herbal medicine are found among the Navajo of the Southwestern United States. The Navajo believe that disease is brought on by deliberate transgressions against certain communal taboos, committed because an individual is out of harmony with himself or with nature. A successful treatment is believed to restore harmony through the use of rituals and herbs, often administered as part of a steam bath.

Indian medicine has been extended to some extent into the folk medicine of more recent arrivals in America. Bringing kit bags of herbal ''receipts'' or ''simples,'' immigrant whites and blacks soon realized that many Indian cures were more effective than their own. Some of the old remedies, along with others adopted in the New World, are still popular cough and cold treatments in such rural areas as the Appalachian valleys of western and southern Virginia.

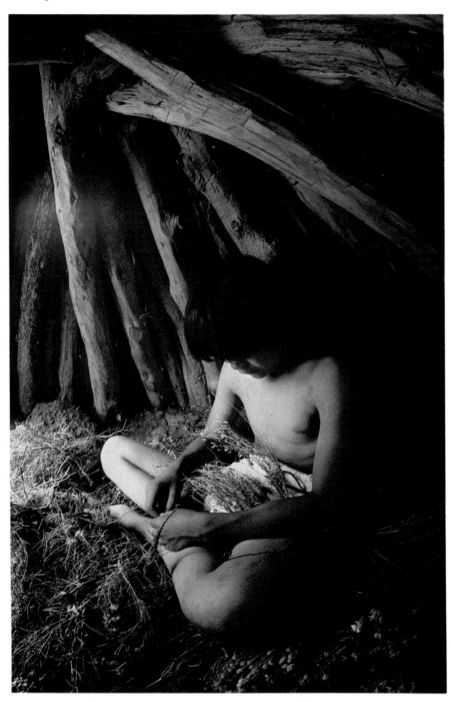

*A Navajo youth with a bad cold waits in a medicine man's hut as preparations begin for his steam bath. Water and herbs will be poured on heated rocks and the medicated steam — like steam from an electrically powered vaporizer — will ease congestion.*

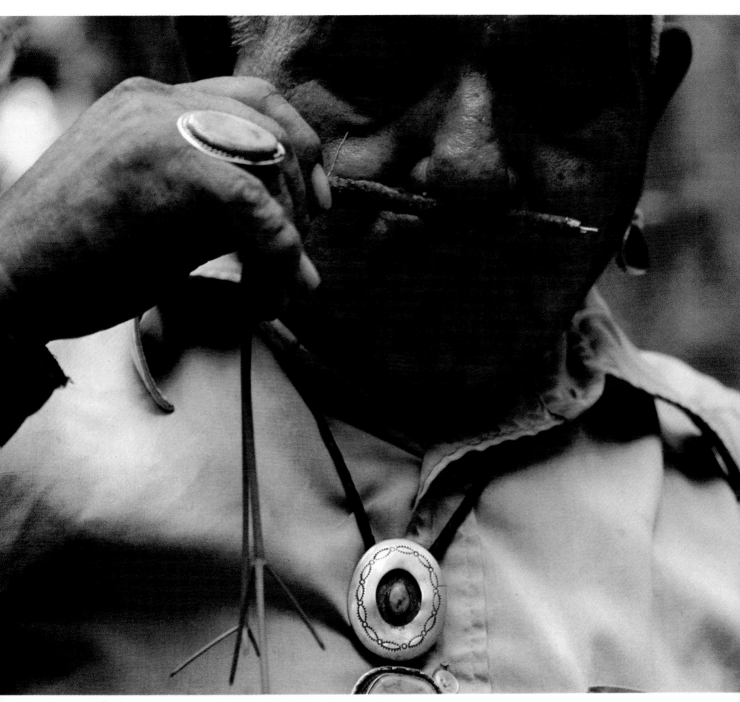

*A Navajo medicine man gives a sniff test to a length of osha root.
As a cold treatment, the root is chewed and its leafy tops are
used in a tea. A variety of parsley that grows wild in the highlands
of the American Southwest, osha is regarded by many Indian
peoples as a wonder drug, which not only cures colds but heals
sores and open wounds and relieves stomach disorders.*

28

*In a morning forage, a Virginia herbalist harvests a full-grown mullein plant and a basketful of mullein leaves. A tea made with the fresh, bitter-tasting leaves seems to help relieve a cough; dried leaves are smoked in pipes or home-rolled cigarettes for the same purpose.*

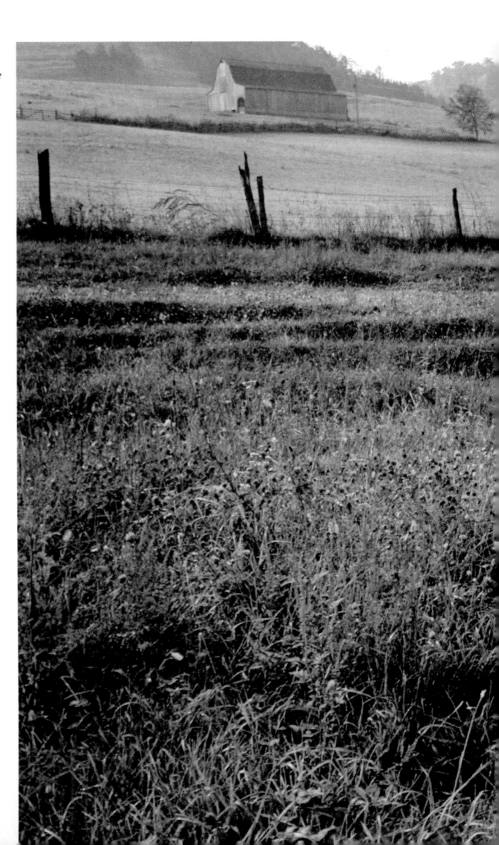

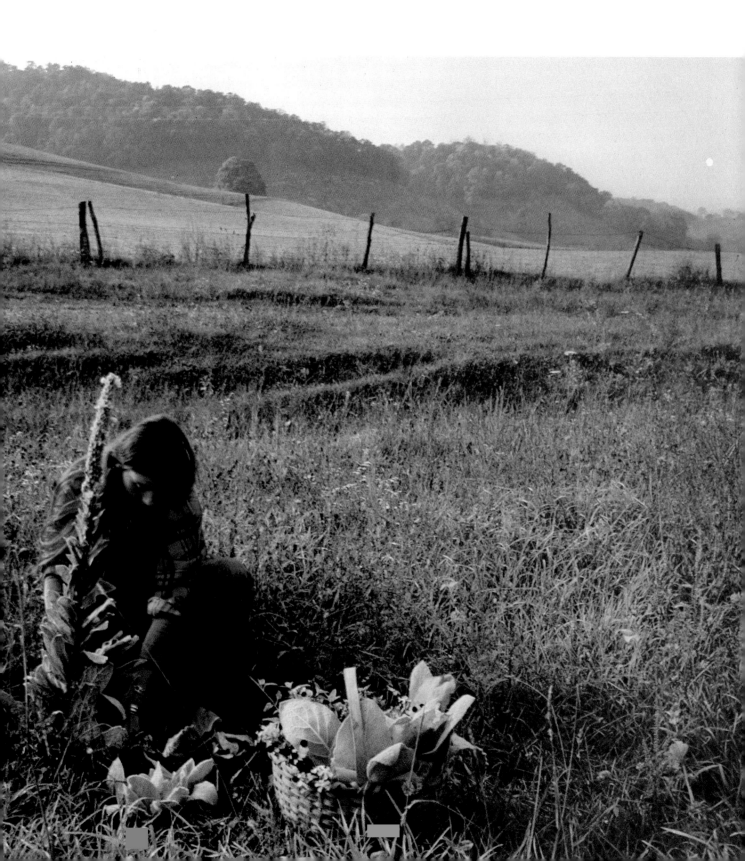

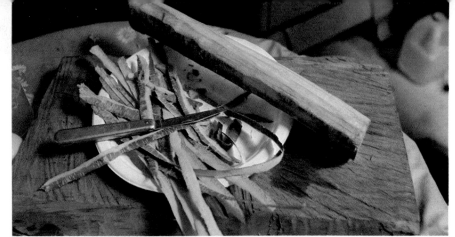

*The inner bark of the wild cherry, a basic ingredient of many homemade cough remedies, is prepared (right) in a rural Virginia kitchen. Slivers of woody outer bark have been pared away, revealing the interior medicinal layer, which has a faint aroma of almonds and an acrid taste.*

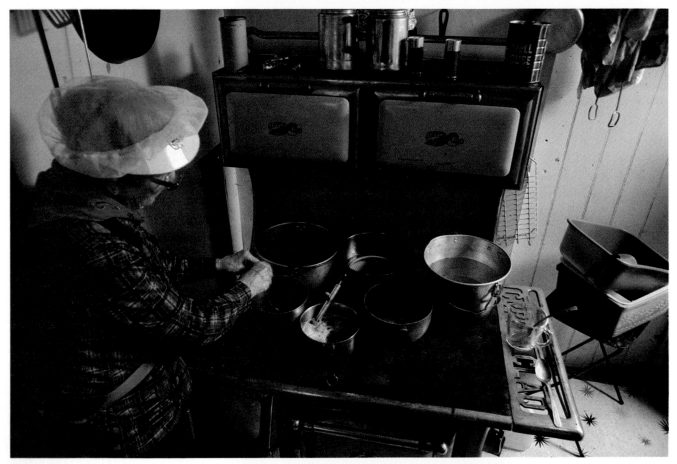

*Keeping an eye on a horehound cough-lozenge mixture simmering on her wood stove, a Virginia herbalist assembles ingredients for a cough syrup. She crumbles bits of wild cherry into a pot (above), and will add red-clover blossoms, tender white-pine twigs, mullein leaves and water. Later she will decant the brew, strained and flavored with honey, into a jar (right).*

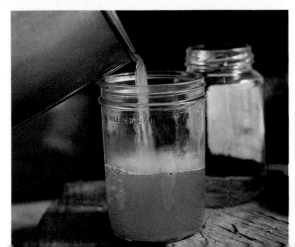

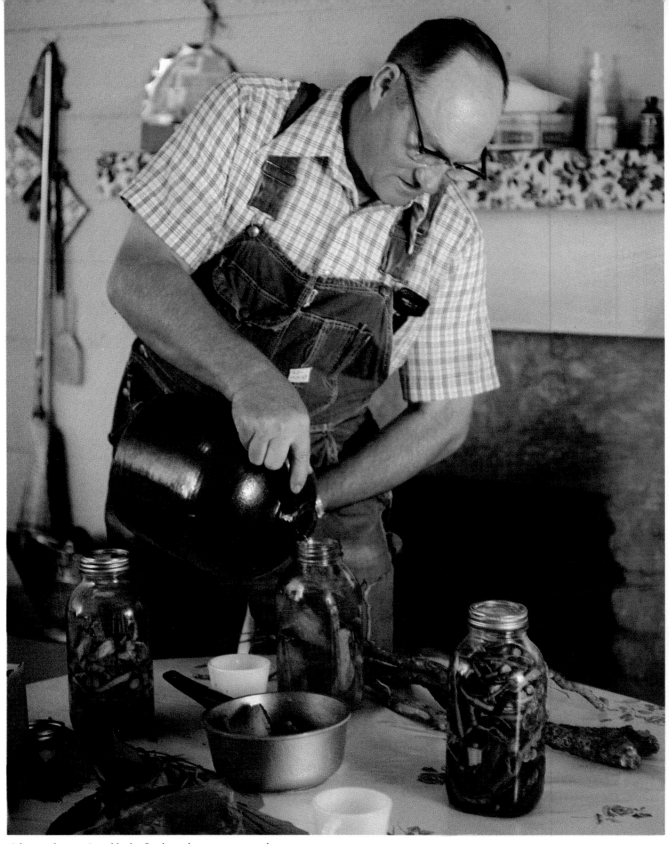

*A home pharmacist adds the final touch — a generous dose
of grain alcohol — to a good-for-what-ails-you tonic based on raw
herbs and barks. Ingredients on the table include wild cherry to
ease nasal congestion, bloodroot to perk up the appetite, ginseng
for energy, and sassafras for flavor. After steeping 24 hours,
the liquid will be strained and set aside for ready use.*

32

# Asia's pin-point remedies

The ancient Chinese healing art of acupuncture, which dramatically relieves pain without the use of drugs, is based on a definition of all life as *ch'i*, or energy. *Ch'i* is described as flowing through the body along imaginary pathways, or meridians. Each meridian has its coupled opposite—another meridian elsewhere in the body, to which its flow of energy is closely related. Thus an organ's condition may be reflected in a remote part of the body.

Good health prevails when the meridian pairs function harmoniously; sickness signals imbalance. Accordingly, treatment consists of stimulating and depressing complementary meridians at a few selected points—more than 1,500 points are designated on the body —until harmony is restored. Needles may be inserted (classic acupuncture), heat introduced (moxibustion, shown on pages 34-35), massage applied, or several techniques used togeher. The choice of therapy depends on the patient's physical and mental state.

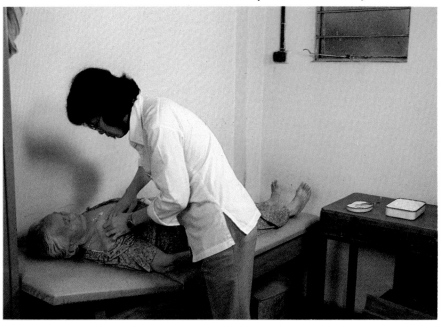

*An acupuncturist at Malaya's Medical Training Institute attends a patient who has a respiratory ailment. Having inserted a needle, he rotates it between thumb and forefinger, constantly questioning the patient on the nature of her sensations.*

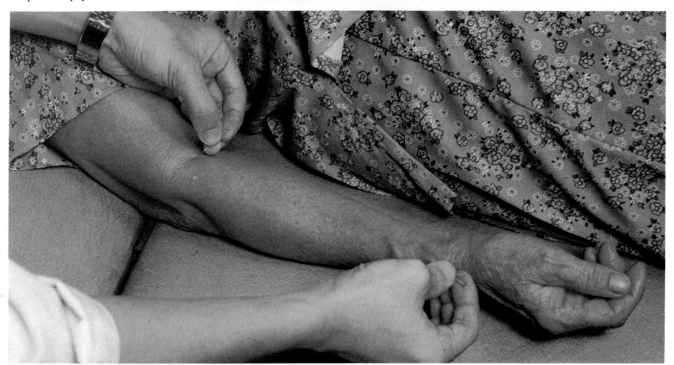

*Continuing the therapy, the physician manipulates needles at two other points. Depending upon the tissue and the sensitivity of the patient, he sets his needles at different depths: In the wrist area, the needles pierce to a depth of about one centimeter; the second needle, inserted near the elbow, goes deeper. Subtle differences in the angles of penetration are also important.*

An assortment of sterilized stainless-steel needles illustrates the so-called filiform type, which are extremely fine in gauge and round in cross section. Used less often are the "three-edge," triangular in section; the "plum blossom," made up of a cluster of five to seven needles; and a technologically sophisticated electrical needle complete with a voltage regulator.

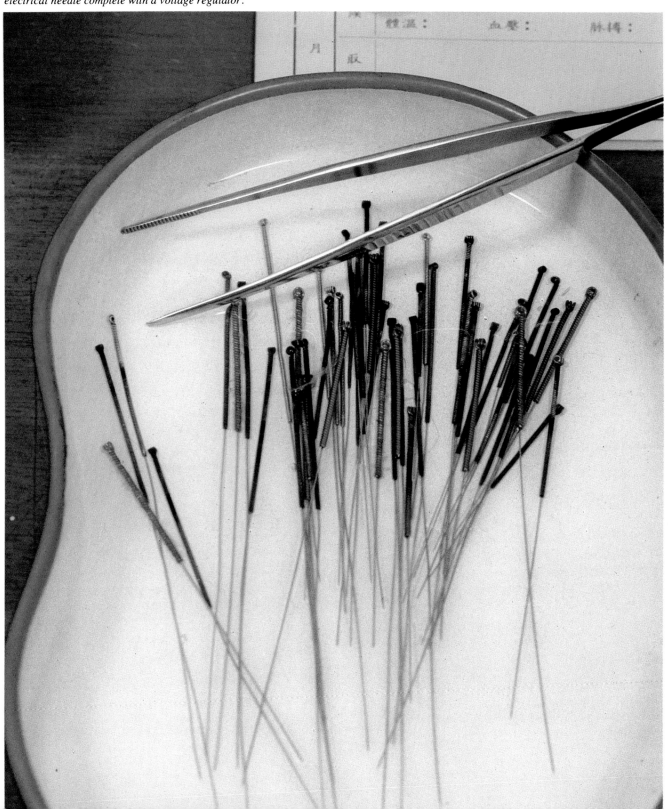

The moxa stick, a roll of powdered wormwood wrapped in rice paper, is a basic tool of moxibustion. The box of 10 eight-inch sticks shown here was commercially prepared in China. Cone-shaped wads of moxa, ranging from the size of a cherry to that of a grape seed, are also prepared by individual practitioners for use as a particular disease requires.

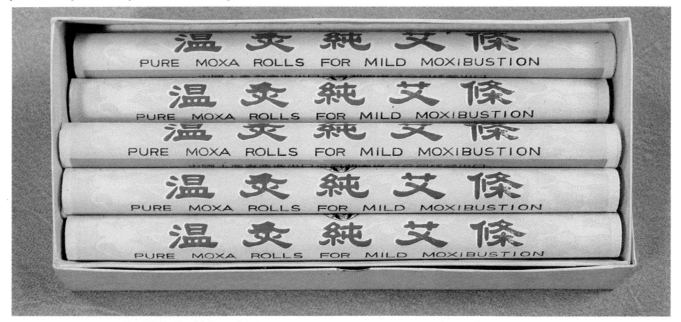

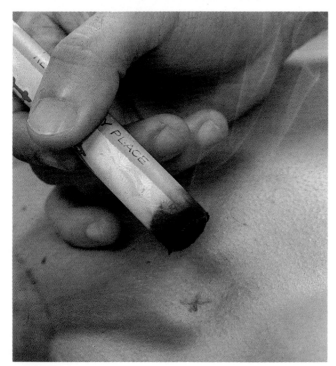

To treat a patient suffering from cough and congestion, a therapist holds a smoldering moxa stick about an inch and a half above a marked acupuncture point on the skin; the point treated here, called Tiantu (meaning ''celestial support'' or ''heaven's gate''), is located on the base of the neck. When the area turns bright pink, the stick is moved to the next point.

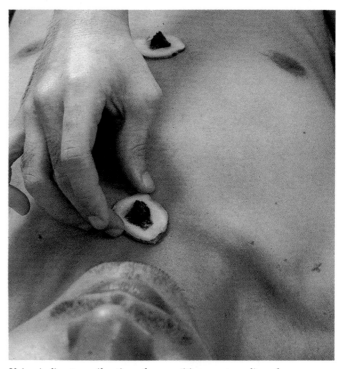

Using indirect moxibustion, the practitioner sets a slice of ginger topped with a burning moxa wad at an acupuncture point. When the patient feels the heat, indicating that the moxa has nearly burned through the ginger, a fresh slice is set in place. The procedure is repeated two or three times. Ordinarily the flesh becomes only pleasantly warm, but blisters occasionally form.

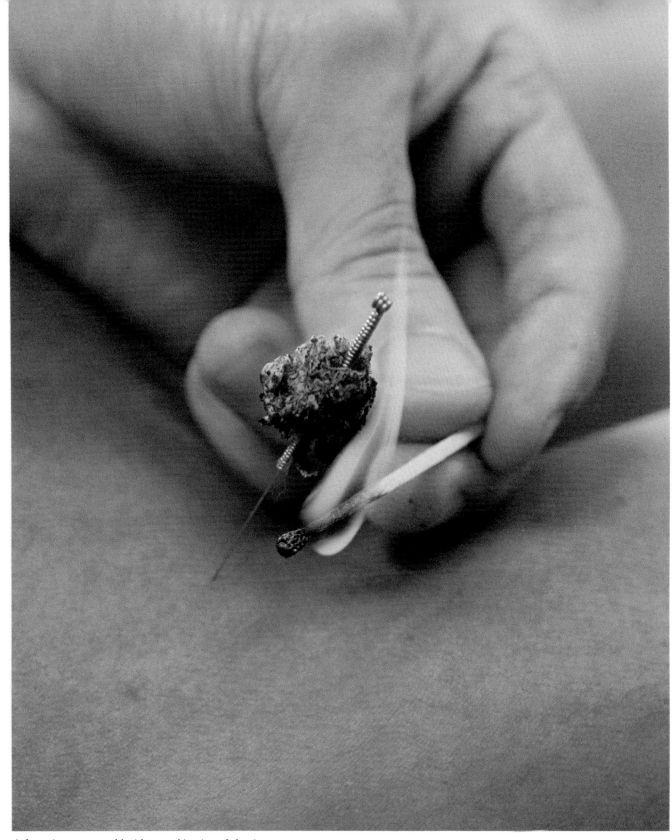

*A therapist treats a cold with a combination of classic
acupuncture and moxibustion, on the theory that their cumulative
effect reaches deeper below the skin. In the procedure above, a
wad of moxa wool is slipped over the needle handle and ignited;
in a more refined version, a piece of paper is fitted onto
the needle beneath the moxa to protect the skin from ashes.*

# CHAPTER 2

# Keeping your defenses up

**Breaking the chain of transmission**
**How interferon rallies the body**
**Fever—both good and bad**
**The cold—partly in your mind?**

Humorist Robert Benchley once addressed himself to the mysterious phenomenon of the common cold. After due deliberation he offered "rules for avoiding the common head cold," among them:

- "Don't breathe through your mouth or nose.
- "Avoid crowds. A good way to avoid crowds is to stay right in your room all day with the door locked.
- "Get plenty of sleep. If you feel drowsy at your work, just put your head over on your desk and take a little nap. Your boss will understand if you put a little sign up by your elbow reading: 'Men asleep here. Cold prevention.'
- "Stay in a temperature of between 60 and 70 degrees. This can be done by jumping on board a train for Palm Beach and lying on the sand for a month or so.
- "Don't dose up with patent medicines and nostrums. A sitz-bath of rock-and-rye twice a day ought to be all the medicinal treatment you will need.
- "Eat a balanced diet. No proteins, no starches, no carbohydrates. Just a good steak and lyonnaise potatoes and asparagus now and then during the day.
- "No exercise. Exercise just stirs up the poisons in your system and makes you a hot-bed of disease. Sit, or lie, as still as possible and smoke constantly.
- "If you think you have caught a cold, call in a good doctor. Call in three good doctors and play bridge.
- "And, above all, don't catch cold."

Benchley's bits of wisdom were scarcely less practical than the cherished notions of cold prevention held by your grandmother—and by many physicians, for that matter—until fairly recently. Everyone swore by some pet theory about the causes of colds and some pet remedy for avoiding them. Most such ideas could be backed up with the testimonial of an individual who had not had a cold in 30 years. If the method did not work for the next person, it was probably the failure of the cold sufferer, not of the method.

In 1966 a United States drug manufacturer listed the advice that Americans passed along to each other as cold gospel. Some of the remedies were daily regimens; others were to be taken at the first inkling of a cold: Eat an apple every night. Drink hot beer with camphor. Chew raw, seasoned peanuts. Eat garlic buds and vinegar pickles. Drink buttermilk and soda water. Sniff glycerin, rose water and myrrh. Wear an onion poultice. Visit a chiropractor. Avoid eating wheat or rye.

British home remedies for colds seem to have been even more fanciful. The Common Cold Unit in Salisbury, England, once catalogued the unsolicited suggestions it had received from helpful citizens. Advice to the unit's scientists included the following recommendations for treating nose infections: Sniff pepper, snuff or cinnamon. Wash the inside of the nose with cod-liver oil, salt water, cream or glycerin. Inhale ammonia or eucalyptus vapors.

British prescriptions for preventive hygiene included: Get plenty of sunshine. Wash handkerchiefs with special detergents. Rub socks with onions daily. Expose the naked body to the cooling breezes of an electric fan for 15 minutes a day.

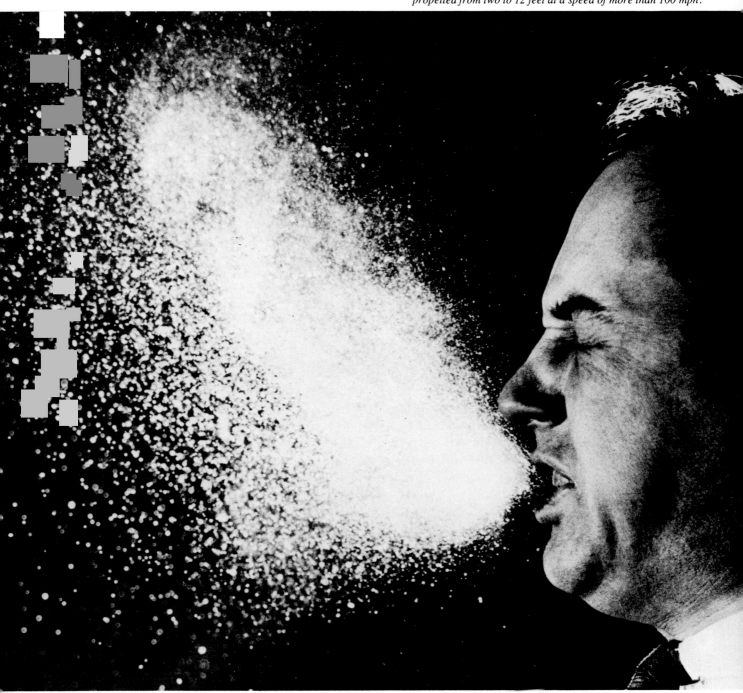

*A classic photograph of a sneeze in eruption, made by Professor Marshall W. Jennison of the Massachusetts Institute of Technology in a 1/30,000-second exposure, has scientific as well as dramatic value. By analyzing such photographs, Jennison determined that a single blast contains over 4,500 droplets, propelled from two to 12 feet at a speed of more than 100 mph.*

Special diets to reduce the incidence of colds contained large doses of onion soup, garlic, carrots or hot lemonade; others banned salads in the fall and winter months. Among the miscellaneous treatments proposed were: Rub the body with petroleum jelly. Smoke tobacco several times a day. Wear a gas mask for an hour daily. Take up fencing. Grow a luxuriantly thick mustache. Stand on the head underwater. Rub naphtha spirits on the scalp. Practice mental concentration, especially on mathematics.

Unfortunately, virtually none of these curatives take into account the fact that viruses are what cause colds. Nor do the remedies allow for the reality that avoiding colds is largely a two-stage process: breaking the viral chain of transmission from one person's respiratory tract to another's, and keeping the body healthy enough to prevent viruses from prospering when they do show up. The first stage offers the better protection: Avoid the avoidable routes of viral transmission. This is simple in theory but difficult in practice.

**Human beings and cold viruses—made for each other**

Without the presence of humanity, the viruses that cause the common cold would have disappeared long ago. No other creature in nature, with the occasional exception of the chimpanzee, can give aid and comfort to these viruses. (Other animals have plenty of other viruses, including some that cause coldlike symptoms, but most of them are so highly specialized that they are incapable of infecting humans.)

Human beings not only give cold viruses a warm welcome, but may continue to play host to them even when all signs of illness have disappeared. From 1974 through 1978, crew members of the Amundsen-Scott (South Pole) Station, after months of isolation from all outside contact each winter, suddenly came down with colds. Researchers found live virus stored in the nasal passages of healthy camp personnel who showed no apparent symptoms of infection. In these healthy carriers, the virus was held in check, but at certain times of the year it was passed on to other hosts, and there it flourished.

Because climate and isolation at the South Pole stations are unique, the researchers were unable to say for certain wheth-

## The eccentric Macfadden method

Of the myriad remedies offered to cold sufferers through the ages, few match the imaginative eccentricities of those set forth in a 1926 book called *Colds, Coughs and Catarrh*. It prescribes a no-nonsense regimen including daily enemas, nude outdoor "air baths," meals of oranges and water—and the bedtime treatment pictured at right, in which the cold victim has wound damp sheets around various parts of her body.

This strategy was the invention of Bernarr Macfadden, a self-proclaimed "physical culturist" and a successful publisher of magazines and newspapers. Macfadden, who kept himself in undeniably fine shape, celebrated his 81st birthday by skydiving—for the first time. He died in 1955, at the age of 87.

Macfadden believed that colds are caused by an accumulation of poisons in the body; the enemas and spartan diet were intended to drive out the toxins. "Eating when the body is not in condition to handle food," he warned, "is overeating." Macfadden also praised the wet-sheet treatment as a "powerful eliminator"—a claim he never explained.

er healthy carriers spread colds elsewhere. However, the findings may force rethinking of virologists' long-held belief that cold sufferers stop giving off infectious viruses about the time they start feeling better.

If, as the present evidence indicates, cold viruses spread mainly from people who are sniffling and sneezing, cold prevention is somewhat simplified—transmission of the viruses becomes a bit easier to interrupt. Most cold viruses are transmitted by personal contact with a virus shedder or with a shedder's immediate environment. Contact includes an obvious form of touching—handshaking—and the handling of such objects as handkerchiefs, pencils, telephone receivers, drinking glasses or door knobs that shedders have contaminated with virus-laden mucus.

Cold viruses get into the body mainly through the nose and eyes. Rubbing virus-contaminated fingers in the nose or eyes readily transplants the infectious agent. Oddly, the mouth is only a secondary portal for cold viruses. The type that causes more colds than any other, the rhino virus, does not seem to

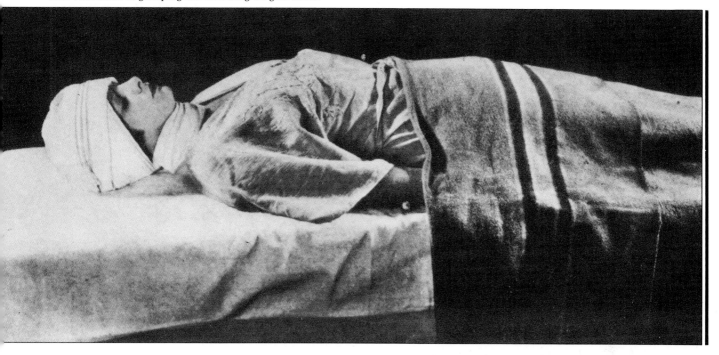

*Among the treatments suggested in a medically dubious 1926 book on colds by physical-fitness zealot Bernarr Macfadden were cold packs around the throat and head, to be wrapped as in this picture. Macfadden advised his readers to avoid colds by breaking such bad habits as gossiping and attending bargain sales.*

infect the body by way of that route. In 1961 British scientists of the Common Cold Unit reported an experiment in which they tried to infect volunteers with cold viruses. Of those infected by way of the nose, about a third developed colds; of those given viruses by way of the throat, none got sick. Similar experiments in America later produced the same result. Thus kissing may be less a mechanism of cold contagion than is generally thought.

Direct contact does not require touching, however. Contact extends to the three feet or so over which large droplets of virus-laden mucus from a sneeze or a cough may score a direct hit on a hand or a nasal membrane. If large particles fail to fall on a new victim, on the cold victim or on nearby objects, they settle on the floor within 10 seconds and are seldom of further consequence except to a crawling baby.

But coughing and sneezing—even singing and talking—may also expel very small droplets, particles so tiny that 25,000 of them laid end to end would hardly make an inch. These microscopic particles may waft about in the air for many minutes before landing on some surface. In this aerosol form they may be inhaled in sufficient numbers to start infection in the nose and throat of a healthy individual many feet away. Settled on a surface, where they may remain infectious for several more hours, they can still be picked up on hands, though usually in concentrations too small to have any effect. Good room ventilation is the best means of dispersing such invisible material and thus reducing the chance of infection.

Popular belief has long held that people catch most of their colds by being in the same room with someone who has a cold. It is simple good manners to cover your mouth when you sneeze and cough, and simple good sense to stay out of whispering distance of cold carriers when their nose-blowing, sneezing and coughing are at a peak. Scientific studies have to a large extent borne out the value of these precautions, but they have also shown that such practices defend against only part of the problem.

To get a notion of how much infectious material is smeared about in the immediate environment of a cold sufferer despite ordinary precautions, a researcher at Britain's Common Cold Unit tried a somewhat eccentric experiment. The experimenter, explained the former director of the unit, Sir Christopher Andrewes *(page 142)*, ''rigged up on his nose an apparatus which permitted fluid to trickle out at about the same rate as would occur with a good cold. He used a handkerchief to blow his nose in an ordinary way as necessary. The fluid contained a dye normally hardly visible but fluorescing brilliantly in ultra-violet rays. He spent some hours in a room with other people, playing cards, eating a meal and so on. At the end of the time, the lights were turned off and a U-V lamp revealed the horrible truth: his artificial nose-secretion had got around everywhere—all over his face and clothes, his food, the playing cards.''

Similar discoveries were made by a team of researchers at the University of Virginia. Focusing on the rhino viruses that are responsible for nearly half of all colds, the investigators found that 50 per cent of their adult subjects with colds carried large quantities of virus on their hands and, like the glowing Briton, consistently deposited them on surfaces in their environment. Moreover, the rhino viruses in the subjects' nasal discharge survived for several hours, dry or wet, visible or invisible, on nonporous surfaces and on skin—and they could be transferred to another individual by no more exposure than a 10-second touch.

In a study to see how often people unconsciously put their hands to their noses and eyes, the Virginia researchers concluded that healthy people may play an important, if inadvertent, role in contaminating themselves with cold viruses. The scientists observed seven groups of adults, some in a conference of physicians, others in a Sunday school class. In a typical hour, a third of the subjects touched their noses and a slightly higher proportion put fingers to eyes.

### Breaking the chain of transmission

What is now known about the transmission of cold viruses indicates that some social niceties are not really as useful as they were thought to be. Covering a sneeze, for example, might be as likely to spread certain colds as letting the sneeze explode rudely into the atmosphere. In an uncovered sneeze the viruses are not concentrated in one place; the hand that traps a sneeze, by contrast, is a focal point of infectious materials that can be transferred to an unfortunate victim. But the whole truth is not that simple. Many viruses spread better through the air than by touch, and the cold sufferer cannot be sure what sort of virus he has. In the balance, the conclusion

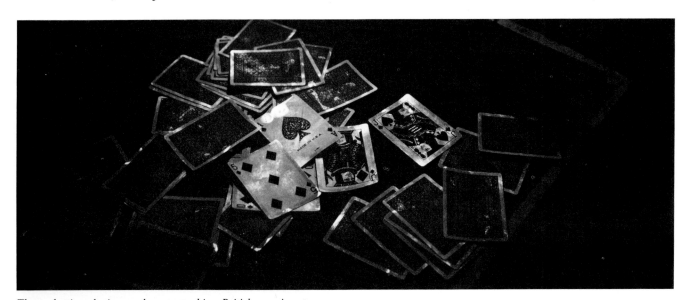

*These glowing playing cards were used in a British experiment to find how a cold sufferer transmits his infection. One player in a bridge game wore a forehead tube that leaked fluorescent dye at about the same rate that a runny nose leaks mucus. Though the player used a handkerchief throughout the game, the glowing spots on the cards indicate heavy contamination.*

is: Anyone with a cold should cover the sneeze, then wash his hands as soon as possible.

Handshaking is another of those courteous gestures that can end up passing around cold germs. Think of a cold sufferer who blows his nose and a few minutes later reaches out a hand in greeting. By now, that hand is a veritable sanctuary for viruses, holding a cold for the next victim. Some experts think it is better manners to keep your hands in your pockets and limit your hearty greetings to words.

Whether to use cloth handkerchiefs or paper facial tissues is another question worth considering in the light of modern knowledge. When handkerchiefs came along as standard equipment for gentlefolk a few centuries ago, they represented a great improvement in hygiene over earlier nose-blowing manners. As recently as the 16th Century, the great Dutch philosopher Erasmus felt it necessary to warn in his *Little Book of Good Manners for Children,* ''To blow your nose on your hat or clothing is rustic, and to do so with the arm or elbow befits a tradesman.'' His advice: ''It is proper to wipe the nostrils with a handkerchief, and to do this while turning away, if more honorable people are present.''

Erasmus was closer to the truth than he knew. Handkerchiefs, researchers can now confirm, do a reasonably good job of trapping nasal discharge and the viruses that may go with it. So do face masks, particularly if they are the very tight-fitting—and uncomfortable—type used by surgeons in operating rooms. The material of which these crude breath filters are made is also important. Researchers at the University of Virginia noted that cotton, paper tissues and other relatively porous fabrics have the further advantage of absorbing and, over several hours, apparently neutralizing viruses that are still alive and raring to go on harder-finished fabrics such as nylon and polyester, which are less absorbent than cotton or paper.

A problem with even the best handkerchief is what to do with it once it is used. As the advertising slogan of a facial tissue manufacturer said, ''Don't put a cold in your pocket.'' A handkerchief becomes a little more contaminated each time it is used—and so do other objects it touches, including the hand that wields it. Paper tissues, discarded after a single

use, have the advantages of porous fabric while offering fewer opportunities for passing viruses on. Experimental tissues impregnated with virus-killing chemicals are being tested on crew members of an isolated South Pole research camp *(pages 144-145)* in hope of making the tissues even more effective than they are now.

The one thing that is clear is that trying to break the chain of transmission in colds is an important part of cold prevention—not only for the cold sufferer but for the healthy person as well. Interrupting the transmission of the virus can never provide full proof against colds by itself, but it can help—and it can also help block the spread of other, potentially more serious, infections. The effort required is small; the techniques are those of elementary sanitation. When anyone in your family has a cold, insist that the other members protect themselves with frequent hand washings, especially after spending time in the same room with the victim. The responsible cold sufferer should do the same (youngsters can be taught the habit at an early age). Also, do whatever is needed to promote air circulation in the house; stuffy interiors do everyone a disservice. Provide the sick person with an ample supply of facial tissues and a place to deposit them: A paper bag reserved for tissues only is the most efficient ar-

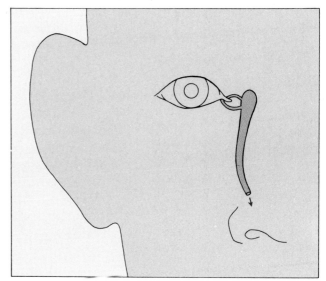

*A tube called the nasolacrimal duct, running from the inside corner of the eye to the nose, normally drains off the unshed tears that constantly cleanse and moisten the eyeball. The duct can also be a source of infection: Cold viruses that are picked up on the fingers may be rubbed into or deposited on the eye and then washed along with the tears to the nose.*

rangement. Members of the household should use separate face soaps, towels and wash cloths.

Some other precautions often recommended may not help as much as many people think. Because the most important cold viruses—the rhino type—do not seem to enter the body through the mouth, separate or disposable drinking glasses and dinnerware may be less valuable protection against colds than separate towels. However, other kinds of virus and bacteria may infect by way of the mouth, and hands that touch a drinking glass may pick up viruses that are transmitted later on to the nose or eyes. For these reasons glasses and dinner-

ware should not be overlooked as transmitters of disease.

Perhaps the most important commandment of anticold sanitation is: Keep hands away from nose and eyes. The nose and eyes are, after all, the principal route of attack a cold virus can take. Anyone who could keep all viral invaders away from these portals might never catch a cold.

### The bodyguards

When hygienic prevention efforts fail, as they sometimes must, the body itself takes over to protect against the consequences. A cold virus that finds its way into the vulnerable

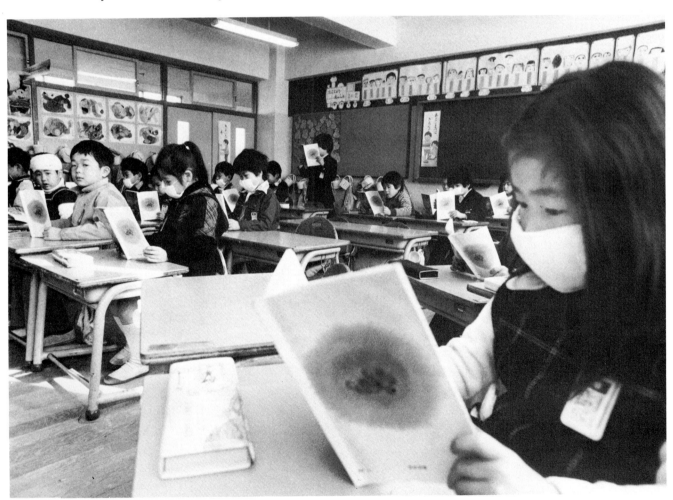

*Tokyo children wear face masks during a cold epidemic in the hope of containing the contagion. Widely adopted in Japan during the 1918-1919 influenza pandemic, the masks are now used by young and old alike, even after a cold has been contracted. Said one mask wearer: ''There are people all around you and you don't want to give your cold to others. It's only courteous.''*

nose encounters various defenses in the body's respiratory, blood and nervous systems *(pages 54-61)*. Some of these defenses are mechanical, some chemical. Some of them work locally at the site of infection; some involve the body as a whole. Many overlap one another in the protection they give. Most of the time these loyal bodyguards function so quietly and anonymously that it is easy to forget their existence. Yet, in their unspectacular ways, they work 24 hours a day repulsing or disarming the millions of persistent and extremely varied disease agents that invade the body. The stakes entrusted to these defenders are high—literally a matter of life or death in some cases. Even cold viruses might attack heart, lungs and brain if they were allowed to operate unopposed.

On the front line of defense in the respiratory system are the coarse nostril hairs, several hundred of which stand at the entrance of the nose to screen out large airborne particles and droplets of moisture that may carry disease agents. Immediately beyond the hairs is the nasal mucous membrane. A sort of multilayered internal skin, the membrane contains blood vessels, nerves and mucous cells, the last secreting both the viscid, normally clear substance called mucus and a chemical activator, or enzyme, called lysozyme. The mucus gathers up viruses, bacteria, dust, pollen and other irritants as they enter the nose and throat. If the intruders are bacteria, the mucus succeeds in destroying some on the spot through the action of the lysozyme. As for viruses and other irritants, the mucus simply wraps them in its enveloping blanket, suspending them away from the surface of the membrane so that they remain harmless.

To clear the debris away, the top layer of cells of the mucous membrane in the nose and in some parts of the throat is equipped with many millions of filaments called cilia, invisible to the naked eye but looking something like a field of grain when they are observed under an electron microscope *(pages 46-47)*. The cilia move back and forth in sweeping waves, each sweep advancing the mucus blanket through the nasal passageways toward the back of the mouth. There, the mucus normally leaves the upper respiratory tract and enters the digestive tract, where it is eventually de-

## Common sense from Dr. Franklin

For centuries, medical wisdom asserted that colds were brought on by either cold weather or moisture. In the late 1700s, however, the statesman, scientist and homespun philosopher Benjamin Franklin took a hard, empirical look at this orthodox view and came up with some heretical conclusions about the causes of colds.

"Travelling in our severe Winters," he recalled, "I have suffered Cold sometimes to an Extremity only short of Freezing, but this did not make me *catch Cold*." He was equally skeptical about the connection between colds and damp. An enthusiastic swimmer, he noted: "I have been in the River every Evening two or three Hours for a Fortnight together, when one should suppose I might imbibe enough of it to *take Cold* if Humidity could give it; but no such effect followed." His skepticism as to the role of humidity in causing colds was further reinforced by his knowledge of the human body. Atmospheric dampness, he argued, "of itself can never by a little Addition of Moisture hurt a Body filled with watry Fluids from Head to foot."

Having disproved the prevailing view to his own satisfaction, Franklin made a shrewd guess at the true mechanism of contagion. Though he wrote at a time when the infectious nature—or even the existence—of microscopic disease organisms had not yet been recognized, his guess came close to a modern description of the process. Colds were caused, he suggested, by "the frowzy corrupt Air from animal Substances, and the perspired matter from our Bodies." As usual, he backed his theory with concrete observation. "People often catch Cold from one another," he wrote, "when shut up together in small close Rooms, Coaches, &c. and when sitting near and conversing so as to breathe in each others Transpiration."

Franklin's solution to the cold problem? Plenty of fresh air—a remedy he championed with evangelistic fervor. In the fall of 1776, future President John Adams wrote in his diary that, when he shared a room at an inn with Franklin, the sage of Philadelphia insisted on throwing open the window. Adams reported that when he protested that the chill night air would surely cause a cold, Franklin happily embarked on "a harrangue, upon Air and cold and Respiration and Perspiration"—an explanation so lengthy that Adams fell asleep in midsentence, with the window still open.

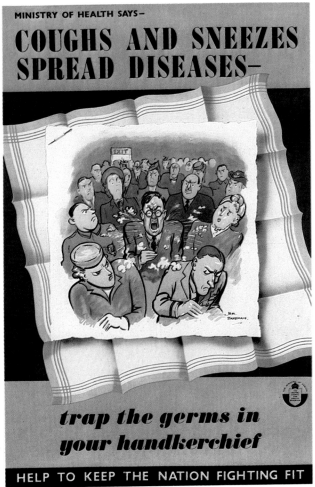

*A British poster exhorts the nation to keep in fighting trim for World War II by using handkerchiefs. Later research found that the exhortation was oversimplified. A handkerchief does block large droplets expelled in coughs and sneezes, but it cannot trap smaller ones; at best, it only redirects them off to the side.*

stroyed. The trachea and part of the larynx—the lower and upper parts of the air passage to the lungs—are also lined with cilia, but here the cilia push the mucus upward and away from the lung area to join the nasal discharge that flows into the digestive tract.

Researchers have found that the rate of ciliary motion, and thus the rate of mucus clearance, varies considerably from person to person. The sweeping action can also speed up or slow down in the same person as the result of changes in body chemistry, often induced by substances that are eaten, drunk or inhaled—tobacco and alcohol, for example, slow the waving cilia. Ten minutes from nostril to throat is about the average time needed to move out a particle, viruses included, in a healthy individual. In people with sluggish cilia, the trip may take longer than 30 minutes. A direct relationship between the speed of clearance and a person's resistance to disease remains to be proved, but slow clearance seems to increase the chance that a virus can penetrate the mucus and form an infectious attachment. Some specialists advise anyone plagued by recurrent colds to cut back on alcohol and tobacco for a few months to see if any improvement in resistance results.

**How interferon rallies the body**

Viruses that do succeed in penetrating the mucus and attaching themselves to membrane cells set off a series of reactions called immune responses. Working through a variety of cell types and unique chemical substances, the immune responses act to isolate the trouble, whatever it may be, and prevent it from spreading. The responses divide into two broad categories of activity: one nonspecific, attacking whole classes of enemies, the other specific, keyed to attack a very narrow range of adversaries with powerful effect. Although each specific agent works against only a single kind of invader, all the specific agents together cover a vast range of potential enemies.

The first nonspecific troubleshooter to arrive is an antiviral substance called interferon. At the onset of a cold, the infected cells release interferon into fluids of the mucous membrane and it begins to make surface contact with still-healthy cells nearby. When a virus later attaches itself to one of these "prepared" cells, it finds the host cell less submissive to the invasion. Interferon has somehow induced the cell to produce antiviral chemicals that keep it from collaborating with the enemy; the cell thus does not make more viruses, as body cells do when overwhelmed by a virus invader *(page 23),* and it remains fully capable of producing its own materials in normal fashion.

Viruses vary greatly in their propensity to spur cells into producing interferon, and they also vary considerably in their susceptibility to interferon blockage. The extent of interferon's role in defending the nose and throat against colds and in limiting their duration is not precisely known, and scientists presume that the answers, when found, will vary for each group of viruses.

After several days of holding the line in lonely battle, the cells and interferon begin to get some help from another nonspecific defense, inflammation. The results of the inflammation process are familiar to every cold sufferer: redness, heat, swelling and occasional pain inside the nose. The normally pink, shiny surface of the mucous membrane turns an almost fiery red and the sensations are the common symptoms of a cold—a runny, stuffy nose, often accompanied by a mildly sore throat.

This onset of discomforts is usually the first overt signal to the victim that a cold is "coming on." The fact is that the cold is already there. The burgeoning discomfort is less a mark of viral damage than of the body's first steps to conquer the virus—the invasion, though destructive, was essentially painless. The cold sufferer feels fine while being attacked by infection, discovers he has "just" caught a cold at the point when his body is beginning to cure it, and feels miserable mainly because his body is making him well.

The inflammation begins immediately after the incubation stage of a cold, when membrane cells, such as the mast cell pictured on page 58, spill substances known as mediators into the tiny spaces surrounding the cells. Among the first of these mediators to be released is histamine, which sets off a powerful local reaction almost immediately—it directs nearby blood vessels to expand and thus increase the flow of warm blood to the damaged area. This process produces the redness and heat of inflammation.

The dilation of the blood vessels also helps increase their permeability, much as stretching a stocking enlarges the spaces between the threads. Through these spaces seep blood plasma (essentially blood fluid minus its red and white cells) and some blood chemicals, including a series of defensive compounds known collectively as complement *(page 51).* The fluid floods tissue spaces within the mucous membrane. This infusion of liquid into the tissues causes them to swell, narrowing the nasal passages. The swelling of tissues with fluids to narrow nasal passages is popularly known as congestion, a word that is frequently misunderstood. It does not mean that the nasal passages become blocked with thickened mucus, nor do the nasal decongestants employed against congestion remove mucus. Their effect is to temporarily reduce swelling of the tissues surrounding the passages, returning them to normal size and giving the mucus more room to move out.

As the nasal tissues swell, mucus-secreting cells increase their production, causing an excess of moisture on the surface of the passages. Some of the mucus, unable to make its way up through the constricted nasal passages, has no place to go and must drip out the front of the nose—and the nose begins to run.

The swelling and destruction of the nasal tissues are likely to impinge on nerve endings in the area, causing them to send impulses to the brain, where they are interpreted as pain. Irritations in the region of the nose and eyes may also send complaints to another site in the brain, setting in motion the almighty sneeze. In a Rube Goldberg sequence of events, the sneeze center of the brain sends a series of commands to the muscles around the lungs that lead to a violent explosion. Mucus-laden air exits primarily from the mouth but also from the nose at speeds exceeding 100 miles an hour and is propelled as far as 12 feet. The sneeze brings temporary help in clearing the area of excess mucus and fluids.

Inflammation and mucus in the pharynx, larynx, trachea and still lower segments of the respiratory system frequently produce coughing, another auxiliary defense mechanism.

Unlike a sneeze, a cough may be either voluntary or involuntary—some coughs are uncontrollable, but others can be initiated by a conscious decision. The cough center of the brain instructs chest and abdomen muscles to tighten and simultaneously orders the glottis, a narrow opening at the top of the larynx, to close. The tightening muscles squeeze the lungs but air cannot escape from them because the larynx is shut. Consequently, air pressure builds up in the lungs until the glottis opens suddenly; then trapped air rushes upward and out explosively, generating the noise known as a cough. The sudden burst of air in a cough helps keep respiratory passages open and prevent infectious mucus from descending into the lower respiratory tract. When for any reason it fails in this task, more serious secondary infections such as bronchitis and pneumonia can follow.

The frequency of cold-associated sneezes and coughs varies enormously from person to person. It depends in part on an individual's normal threshold of irritation. But in the case of coughs, other factors enter in. One, understandably, is the extent to which the individual is exposed to cigarette smoke or other chronic throat irritants. In one study of individuals suffering from rhino virus colds, the daily rate of coughing for male smokers exceeded that of male nonsmokers by more than 3 to 1 on the first day of infection. Coughing by both groups diminished on the fourth day, though the smokers still had slightly the worse of it. Another factor that influences coughing is, for reasons unknown, gender. Female smokers in the study followed a pattern opposite that of males; they coughed less than male smokers on the first day but were coughing more than twice as much and getting worse by the fourth day. At all times they coughed more than nonsmoking females, and the difference grew as the cold wore on.

### Fever—both good and bad

Yet another by-product of inflammation is fever, which appears occasionally in adults as a symptom of a cold, but relatively often in young children. Technically, fever is defined as an elevation of body temperature above the individ-

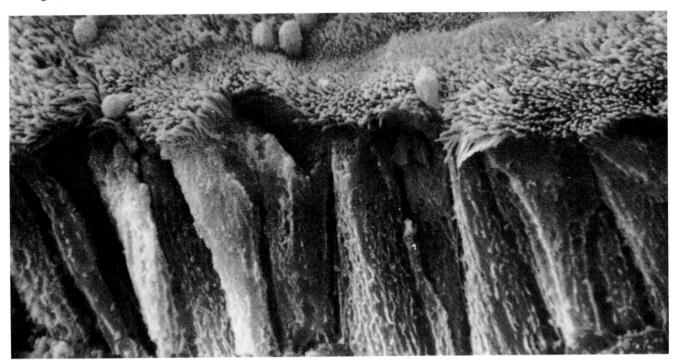

*Cilia, the tiny—less than .0004 inch long—projections that line and clean the respiratory tract, are visible in this scanning electron micrograph and the one at right. Above, in a cross section of nasal tissue, drops of mucus have oozed to the surface of the cilia from the palisade-like cells of the mucous membrane.*

ual's norm, but the facts of fever are far more complex than this simple definition. Though the function of a fever is still obscure and under investigation, the processes that produce it are now clearly understood.

Developing and maintaining body heat, whether within normal ranges or during fever, is an astonishingly complex affair. The heat comes from metabolism, the chemical conversion of food into energy by the body acting as an engine. Some heat needs to be retained to keep the body warm; some must be dissipated to prevent overheating. Temperature regulation requires the body to balance the heat-producing activities of metabolism with those activities that dissipate heat—both the exhalation of heated air through the action of the lungs, and the circulation and cooling of heated blood just beneath the surface of the skin. This balancing act is controlled in a tiny part of the brain called the hypothalamus, which operates certain on-off switches much as an ordinary thermostat in the house does.

When the body is attacked by viruses and counters with the

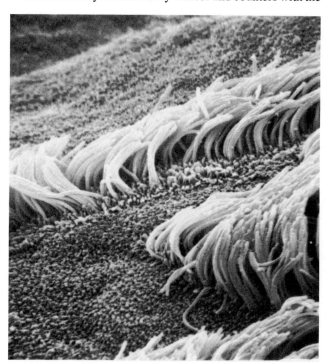

*In this micrograph, more highly magnified than the picture at left, cilia flex in unison at the end of one of their wavelike movements. These strokes, repeated as often as 1,000 times per minute, move mucus along the respiratory tract to the throat, where it is swallowed and dispatched to the stomach.*

first phases of the immune responses, one of the chemical mediators generated is a fever-producing substance called endogenous pyrogen. Released into the bloodstream and carried to the brain, endogenous pyrogen increases the concentration of chemicals called prostaglandins in the hypothalamus. These substances somehow reset the body thermostat, altering the heat-generating and -dissipating relationship to achieve a new and higher norm; the body's metabolism generally accelerates, more food nutrients than usual are used up, and the heart beats faster. At the same time, the blood vessels near the surface of the skin constrict, decreasing circulation and heat loss there, and driving more of the heated blood to the internal parts of the body.

The body often feels chilled during bouts of fever because the brain is calling for a higher temperature than the body has yet reached. The degree of chill experienced is a rough measure of the differential between the higher setting of the brain and the body's lower temperature. Often coincident with chills is shivering. A rhythmic, involuntary muscle contraction, it is the body's attempt to generate heat through motion in order to counteract chills.

The chill phase of a fever is typically followed by a change-over to hot skin and a new series of discomforts. Breathing speeds up, partly to dissipate the increased heat, partly to supply the additional oxygen required by the accelerated chemical processes of metabolism. The sufferer has a dry throat and intense thirst, caused partly by faster breathing, partly by increased evaporation of moisture from overheated skin and partly by damage to the mucous membrane lining the throat. The feverish state ends when the body stops producing endogenous pyrogen and the brain thermostat resets itself downward to normal body temperature. An occasional sign of a rapidly breaking fever is profuse sweating, but the return to normal is more likely to be a gradual, unspectacular affair.

Fever is widely believed to be a dangerous condition that must be overcome for the health of the patient. This idea is fairly recent. Until the end of the 19th Century, physicians considered moderate fever beneficial, a natural response to infection that counteracted the disease. Then opinion sud-

# The right way to use a fever thermometer

One sign that a coldlike illness is more than a cold is fever—a substantial variation from normal temperature. For accurate measurement, you need a fever thermometer—a rectal type for babies, an oral type for anyone more than three years old.

Both types are specially designed to hold their readings—the column of mercury goes up but will not go back down unless you force it to. This one-way movement of the liquid is caused by a constriction at the bulb exit. Thus, to use the thermometer, you must first force mercury past the constriction back into the bulb by shaking *(right)*. For a true oral measurement, wait 20 minutes after eating or drinking anything hot or cold; then place the bulb under your tongue, turn it, and hold it in place for at least three minutes with lips closed. Because the mercury column is very thin, it is impossible to see unless the thermometer is held at an angle that allows the glass to magnify it *(below)*.

**SHAKING DOWN**
*Grasp the thermometer firmly at the end opposite the bulb and shake it hard with quick downward snaps of the wrist (above, right) until the column of mercury falls below the 95° F. mark.*

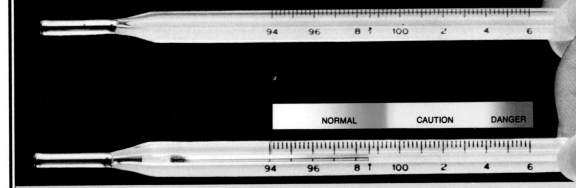

NORMAL          CAUTION     DANGER

**READING THE THERMOMETER**
*Hold the thermometer in good light and rotate it slowly between your fingers; an incorrect position (top) may be only a few degrees of rotation away from the correct one (bottom), at which the band of mercury is clearly visible. Though 98.6° F. is often cited as normal, individuals vary and any reading in the*

*green range above can be considered normal. An elevated temperature (yellow) usually indicates illness more serious than a cold. Consult a physician when a reading rises above 102° in an adult (above 103° in a child) or persists more than three days. Consult a doctor immediately if any fever exceeds 104° (red).*

denly reversed, a change that coincided with the discovery of drugs capable of reducing fever. Now the pendulum of medical opinion seems to be swinging back, for recent research indicates that the ancient view of fever as beneficial may be correct after all. Most of these studies have been done on animals and on isolated tissue in laboratories, and the findings and conclusions have sometimes conflicted with one another.

In experiments on rabbits, investigators found that those that developed fevers as a reaction to a bacterial infection were more likely to survive than those that did not have fevers. And in another study, piglets were better able to fight a gastrointestinal virus when their temperatures were artificially raised above normal.

Some researchers speculate that fever improves the body's defenses by promoting the activity of germ-fighting cells and by improving the effectiveness of interferon.

High fever can be hazardous for many, however. It may dangerously increase heart rates in the elderly or in sufferers from heart and blood-vessel diseases; it can provoke convulsions in young children; it can slow the ability to concentrate; in certain people it can bring on delirium; and in victims of herpes infection a fever may trigger the recurrence of fever blisters.

Of course, fever is an important indicator of infection. In the case of the common cold, a high fever may signal a more serious illness that warrants a doctor's attention.

Whenever fever accompanies a cold, body temperature should be monitored regularly *(left)*—at least three times a day in children and in adults who fall into high-risk categories. A written record of the readings can reveal a pattern that helps the doctor diagnose complications.

## White blood cells to the defense

Viruses that manage to get past the local mechanical defenses, the blocking effects of interferon and the various inflammatory responses must tangle with a range of defenses generated by the white cells of the blood. White cells are one of the most important components of the blood, though outnumbered by red cells 500 to 1. In contrast to the red cells, which are reddish in color, uniform in structure and constrained to a single role—the transport of oxygen—white cells are essentially colorless and of several distinct types and functions. They are charged with the overall responsibilities of defending the body against disease and disposing of sick or dead cells.

Some white cells are agents of nonspecific immune response, identifying foreign materials they chance to encounter and consuming them; they are also the producers of the fever-causing endogenous pyrogen. Others are so specialized as to protect the body against a single type of viral challenge; some of these are the white cells that give a person immunity against reinfection by the same virus. Each type depends in some way on the cooperation of one or more other types to carry out its own functions.

Two of the most important cold-fighting white cells are the monocytes and the lymphocytes. The monocytes are manufactured in the bone marrow, and during the early part of their life cycle they enter the bloodstream and circulate there. Then they leave the blood and enter the tissues, where they undergo physical change. They enlarge and their internal structures become more complex, transforming them into macrophages, literally "big eaters." These cells are rather slow moving and they account for only 3 to 8 per cent of the white-cell population in the blood of a healthy person. Nonetheless, they more than make up for their usually modest presence by being able to divide and multiply when needed. They also have voracious appetites; each aptly named big eater can devour as many as 100 viruses before being sated.

After devouring the invader, the big eater becomes more active—it moves faster and divides more often. It also somehow indicates the identity of its captive to nearby cells of another major type of cold fighter, the lymphocyte, so that the lymphocyte can attack similar viruses more effectively. It is the lymphocyte that is the central actor in conferring specific immunity, that is, resistance to a particular virus.

Specific immunity is a highly complex set of interrelationships and responses that are still far from understood. Some basic outlines are, however, becoming clear. The first generations of lymphocytes are formed in the bone marrow and subsequently develop into two distinct types, known as T cells and B cells. Each of these lymphocytes is sent into the world with its surface so constituted chemically that it can respond to only one of the foreign agents that may enter the body. Some of the cells migrate to the thymus, a small gland located just under the breastbone, where they mature into T cells. The B cells apparently mature in the bone marrow.

Both T and B cells reside principally in the body's lymphoid tissues, lumps that are found under the arms, on the neck just behind the ears, and in the groin, as well as in the tonsils, adenoids and spleen. From these scattered strongholds, a constant supply of B cells and T cells circulates through the body, keeping vigil for any invader. When either type comes upon an enemy for which it is the prescribed defense, it triggers an immunological alarm that intensifies activity both among its own kind and among all other agents of immunity, general and specific, throughout the body.

## Killer T cells targeted against infection

T cells are the first specific immune response that directly attacks infected cells—the T cells do not go after the virus itself but after the cells infected with it. When the body is in a healthy, uninfected state, vast numbers of T cells inhabit the lymph tissue in various parts of the body. From these stations T-cell patrols go out to monitor the bloodstream and tissues for the presence of infectious invaders. Each T cell is programed to be able to respond to only one type of virus; out of every 100,000 T cells, perhaps only one will be

## An American artist's prescription for Indian-style breathing

During 30 years of sketching and painting the Plains Indians, American artist George Catlin became convinced that they were healthier than city dwellers, and that this was largely because of the way they slept: They breathed, he observed, through the nose. Even babies were nose breathers, for Indian mothers pressed a sleeping infant's lips together if necessary.

"The nostrils," wrote Catlin in 1861, "with their delicate and fibrous linings for purifying and warming the air in its passage, have been mysteriously constructed to stand guard over the lungs." Catlin ascribed not only colds, but also "diseases of the liver, the heart, the spine, and the whole of the nervous system" to nocturnal mouth breathing.

Catlin overstated the importance of tight-lipped sleep, but he had a point. The nose does provide a more effective air-filtration system than the mouth, and some modern-day physicians advise cold sufferers to sleep propped up in bed, a position that tends to keep the nasal passages open — and the mouth shut.

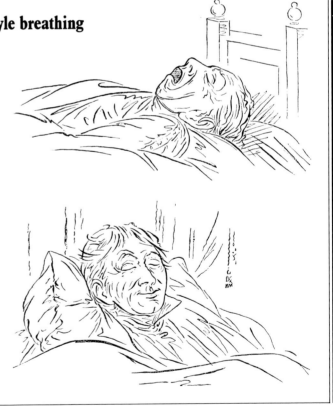

*The troubled sleep of a mouth breather (top) contrasts with the healthful rest of a nose breather (bottom) in sketches by George Catlin. The drawings appeared in Catlin's 1861 booklet, The Breath of Life, a 76-page tribute to the human nose.*

sensitive to the chemical make-up of a given viral invader.

On the second or third day of a cold, when inflammation brings its familiar symptoms, part of the effect of the inflammation is the transporting of hordes of T cells—of all kinds, not just the ones keyed to the invader—to the site of the infection, where big eaters are already at work. There the T cells touch the big eaters, picking up from them the signal that identifies the virus the big eaters have consumed. The relatively few T cells that can react to this signal do so.

T cells activated by the infection, more than B cells, orchestrate the immune responses by secreting substances that perform a number of functions: One substance is a kind of interferon that supplements the interferon produced by infected cells. Another substance attracts all kinds of white cells to the site of the invasion. Still another stimulates big eaters to consume more infected cells. A final substance activates additional T cells that are keyed to the invading virus. But most important, the aroused T cells immediately begin dividing into four kinds of daughter cells, producing great numbers of each kind, all specifically designed to counter the virus that has been identified.

The most important daughter, the killer T cell, is programed to kill outright a cell infected by the virus, thereby interrupting the virus's effort to replicate itself. Another daughter, the helper T cell, is designed to aid B cells in producing antibodies. When antibody production is no longer needed, the third daughter, the suppressor T cell, is signaled to end the activity. Meanwhile, yet another daughter cell, known as the memory T cell, enters the bloodstream. It carries the exact molecular record of the virus that set the whole chain of immune events in motion originally. The memory T cell is thus primed to become the parent of future generations of T cells that, should the same virus return to reinfect the body months or years later, will quash that particular invader.

### Immunity created by B cells

The B cells, meanwhile, also have been activated by contact with the big eaters. They are stimulated, with the assistance of helper T cells, to produce millions of antibodies, the immune system's most sophisticated killers. Antibodies sabotage the invading viruses' weapons, neutralizing the parts of the virus surface that enable the virus to hook onto and enter a host cell. With its attachment sites blocked, the virus is no longer able to invade and take over the host cell.

Antibodies are tailor-made to block the activity of each of the countless different foreign organisms a human may encounter throughout a lifetime. All antibodies have the same basic structural features— four chains of molecules arranged in symmetrical pairs of two light chains and two heavy chains, the whole assemblage joined by a pattern of molecular bridges. Within this basic pattern, a huge number of variations of molecular components occur, making it possible to match an antibody to almost any invader.

Scientists at one time believed that, in fitting perfectly to a single virus, each antibody was totally effective on that virus but of no effect at all on any other. Recently, however, it has become clear that antibodies have relative degrees of affinity to viruses sharing some structural similarity. Thus, not only can an antibody totally block a virus that has made a return visit, but it may also be able to partially block others belonging to the same family of viruses.

In addition to neutralizing a virus's ability to attach itself to a cell, an antibody also contributes to making the invader more susceptible to the scavenger white cells. After an antibody has coated a virus, another part of the antibody surface becomes receptive to the blood substances that are known collectively as complement. Complement includes 11 different compounds that zero in, one after another in a precise sequence, to hit the viral target, where they assist the white-cell scavengers by attracting them to the virus or by helping to destroy the virus.

The combined responses of generalized and specific immunity all work to bring infection to an end. The T cells do much more of this work than the B cells, because they go into action soon after an infection takes hold. The B cells are less effective against a cold because their action depends on the production of antibodies. There are so many types of cold viruses that a person could go on having one type of cold after another, building a reservoir of antibodies in the process,

## The Army's victory over adeno virus

For generations of American military recruits, a special type of heavy cold was one of the perils of basic training. During that two-month period, up to half of the men in a typical batch of trainees spent time on sick call, fevered and coughing: Epidemics beset military services not only in the United States but in Europe as well. Then, in the 1950s and 1960s, U.S. researchers found that just two types of adeno virus were causing most of the military's cold miseries. The strains seldom affected civilians to the same degree; the scientists theorized that the crowded, stressful conditions of basic training were uniquely favorable to viruses.

Because only two virus types were principally involved—rather than the dozens that may infect civilians—use of vaccines for prevention seemed practical. By 1971 the vaccines were available. Within months after their introduction, the incidence of adeno virus infection among recruits was down by more than 50 per cent.

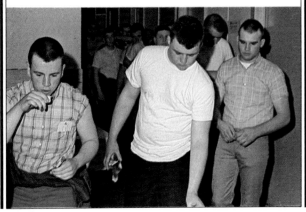

*Shorn but still in civilian dress, recruits at Lackland Air Force Base in Texas await immunization against the adeno viruses that once spawned outbreaks of colds and fever at basic-training camps. Regulations require the recruits to take two aspirin-sized tablets of the oral vaccine during their first 24 hours in camp.*

without ever becoming infected with the same viral strain twice. Besides, the production of enough antibodies to end a disease takes about 14 days, by which time the cold has generally been cured by the other immune responses.

However, antibodies produced by B cells in an earlier cold have a very important effect—they account for, in part, all the weeks and months of good health experienced before the current cold was caught. The antibodies produced too late to help cure an earlier cold have been providing immunity to that kind of virus ever since. The antibodies being produced too late to help in a current cold will do the same for the future.

Thus, if a husband gives his wife a cold, he need not fear catching it back from her—he is immune to that virus, thanks to the work of the B cells' antibodies. In addition, the older an individual gets, the more kinds of cold viruses he is immune to. This conferring of future immunity may be extremely important in keeping the prevalence of colds to its present levels—rhino viruses are a major cause of colds, and immunity to one of the 100-plus types of rhino viruses may mean partial immunity to others, since antibodies are now known to be partially effective against related viruses as well as 100 per cent effective against the target virus.

Some people have immune systems that are less than ordinarily effective, and as might be expected, they suffer extraordinarily from colds. And some studies indicate that people with chronic lung ailments such as bronchitis catch cold easily. Most other aspects of physical condition do not seem to have much effect on vulnerability to this illness; there is no evidence to indicate that vigorous athletes are any less susceptible than people who are chronically ill with heart disease or diabetes.

### The cold—partly in your mind?

One unorthodox area of investigation that intrigues a number of researchers is the possible role of stress in reducing the efficiency of the immune system and opening the way to infections such as colds. Stress in its narrowest physiological sense is a collection of body responses—faster heartbeat and respiration, heightened blood pressure, increased muscle tension, greater hormone output—all designed to gear the body to respond to immediate or anticipated threat. These reactions evolved over the course of human development as a "fight or flight" response, a constructive preparation for the human animal to engage an enemy or to flee from one at all possible speed.

But as the threats to the individuals have become less a matter of physical danger and more one of psychological challenge, the stress mechanisms have ceased to serve their original purpose. Instead, they have become a source of wear and tear for which the body has no productive release. Tension headaches, nervous stomach, aching back and chronic high blood pressure are typical outlets for the threat response today. Some researchers now believe that less obvious ailments, including the common cold, may also be ways by which modern man unconsciously reacts to threats. Certainly, a cold provides an effective rationale for escaping situations that, recognized or unrecognized, can be overwhelming to some individuals.

Pursuing this subject, Richard Totman, an investigator at Britain's Common Cold Unit, set up an experiment aimed at discovering whether there was some link between colds and interruptions in routine social and work activity such as occur after a death in the family, the breakup of a marriage or the loss of a job. He gave 52 volunteers a series of medical tests to determine the cold antibodies in their blood, and then ran them through interviews designed to assess their recent experience of stress and their normal psychological patterns, searching for factors that might indicate neurotic behavior. Each subject was then given nasal drops containing two common rhino viruses. The volunteers were kept isolated to prevent infection from outside sources and from each other for the next 10 days. During this period they were monitored to see who came down with a cold and how severely, as measured partly by their symptoms, partly by the more objective index of how much virus they shed.

When all the information was evaluated, stress factors appeared to play nearly as large a role in determining who got uncomfortably sick as did pretrial levels of antibodies. Totman concluded that psychological factors play a large part in determining whether the body is able to mount an effective defense against a cold. He found also that a person who responded to psychological stress by dropping all normal routines and reducing work and social activity for prolonged periods was far more likely to be vulnerable to infectious assault than the individual who, under the same stresses, went calmly on with the conduct of life. Totman noted one other curious factor that he thinks may play a contributing role in the severity of colds, if not in the contracting of them: Introverts suffered worse symptoms than extroverts, perhaps because they were more given to self-awareness and, ultimately, to self-pity.

In the final analysis colds are almost inescapable. Once you have taken reasonable measures to reduce the opportunities for cold transmission and perhaps to control some of the habits that strain your immune system, you must still resign yourself to existing in a world full of colds and cold sufferers. If you fall victim to a cold, let the severity of the symptoms and your general energy level be your guide in determining how to live with it. If the symptoms are mild and previous bouts with colds have passed uneventfully, there is no medical reason to stay home from your job, school or social activities. Colds do not, after all, spread in epidemics and if you are otherwise healthy your immune system is going to run through its complex choreography of counterattack and recovery without need of extra bed rest or isolation. Indeed, interrupting your normal routines may add strains to the burdens of your cold.

The exception to the rule about holding to usual routines arises if you come into close contact with high-risk individuals—small children, the chronically ill, the elderly. If such contacts are inevitable, break the normal routine to avoid them for the first 48 hours of severe symptoms, if possible. If not, both you and the susceptible parties should be extra-scrupulous in washing, avoiding hand contact and keeping room air circulating freely. These precautions can help block the spread of the virus, which is at its worst during the first two days of symptoms; unfortunately, it spreads for a day or so beforehand, but there is no way to detect that earlier period of contagion. ❃

# The immune system—a cold cure that works

As a superficial infection of the upper respiratory tract, the common cold is just a border incident in the body's wary coexistence with a hostile environment. It is no more than that largely because the defenders of the immune system mobilize to repel the aggressor virus. In a complex sequence of actions directed against both influenza and colds, the body's cells and chemicals slow the infiltration by virus particles, then destroy them and finally create new defenses to block future attacks.

Scientists must deduce some of these actions from experiment. Others, however, can be photographed—using the superb resolution of the electron microscope—in tissues taken from humans and from animals having similar immune systems.

The virus attack begins when a virus particle works its way through the hairlike cilia (*below*) that sweep the respiratory tract, and finds a cell it can infect. As the virus attempts to expand its bridgehead, the target cell *(drawing, right)* releases the chemical interferon, which slows the invasion.

This initial struggle goes on unbeknownst to the human host. But when the infection sets off other immune responses that eventually repel the attack, those defensive actions bring on the familiar runny nose, sneezing and coughing of cold or flu.

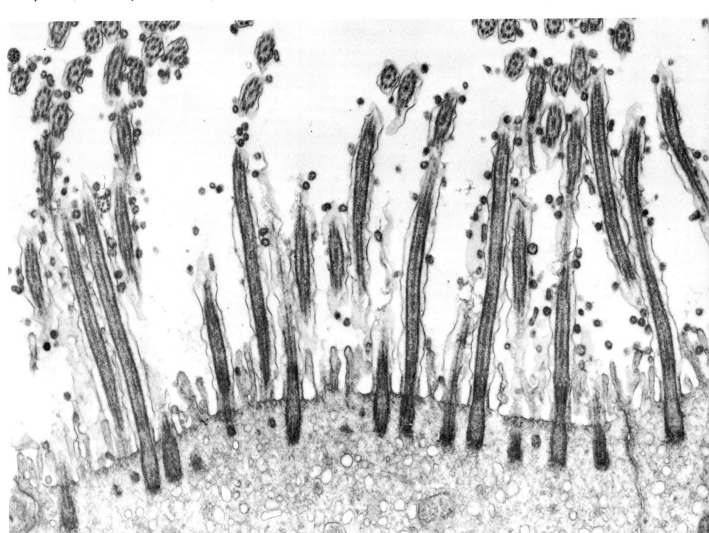

**BREACHING THE FIRST LINE OF DEFENSE**
*The moment of infection is captured in this view of influenza viruses (black particles) as they filter through guinea-pig cilia to reach a cell in the mucous-membrane lining of the respiratory tract. Most infectious invaders are trapped by sticky blobs of mucus supported by the tips of the cilia projections.*

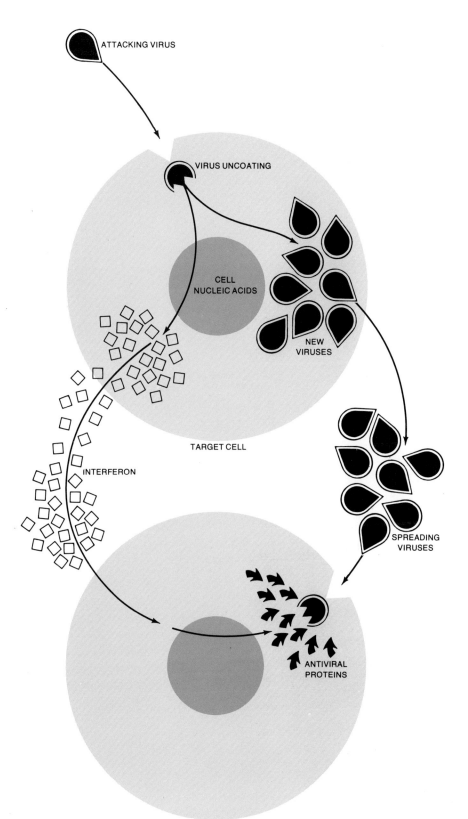

ATTACKING VIRUS

VIRUS UNCOATING

CELL NUCLEIC ACIDS

NEW VIRUSES

TARGET CELL

INTERFERON

SPREADING VIRUSES

ANTIVIRAL PROTEINS

NEIGHBORING CELL

# Interferon's delaying action

### AN ATTACKER MATCHED TO ITS VICTIM
*A cold or flu begins only when a virus encounters a body cell vulnerable to it—one whose surface it matches chemically (indicated here by shapes that fit together). The virus is able to penetrate the wall of such a cell and work its way inside.*

### OVERPOWERING THE CELL MACHINERY
*Once inside the vulnerable cell, the virus sheds its protective coat to expose its core of heredity-controlling nucleic acid. It overpowers the cell's own nucleic acids, seizing control of the cell. Instead of making new host-cell material, the cell is now forced to make viruses.*

### RAISING AN ALARM WITH INTERFERON
*Powerless to resist the destructive orders of the virus, the doomed cell nevertheless is stimulated to produce the substance called interferon. It slips out of the cell and into the surrounding fluid starting about three to four hours after the attack— several critical hours before the new viruses emerge from the original target cell, leaving it in ruins, and seek new cells to attack.*

### ALERTING OTHER CELLS FOR RESISTANCE
*Making contact with the wall of a neighboring cell, the interferon gives the cell a chemical signal that prepares it to make antiviral proteins. These chemicals can block the commands of a virus.*

### STOPPING A VIRUS TAKE-OVER
*The cell is unable to keep one of the new viruses from penetrating it. But its antiviral proteins prevent the cell from obeying the commands of the virus. The cell is thus able to continue making its own proteins, and the virus cannot take over. Unfortunately, interferon is limited in its effect. It may only slow the spread of the infection over the first few days of illness.*

# Launching the counterattack

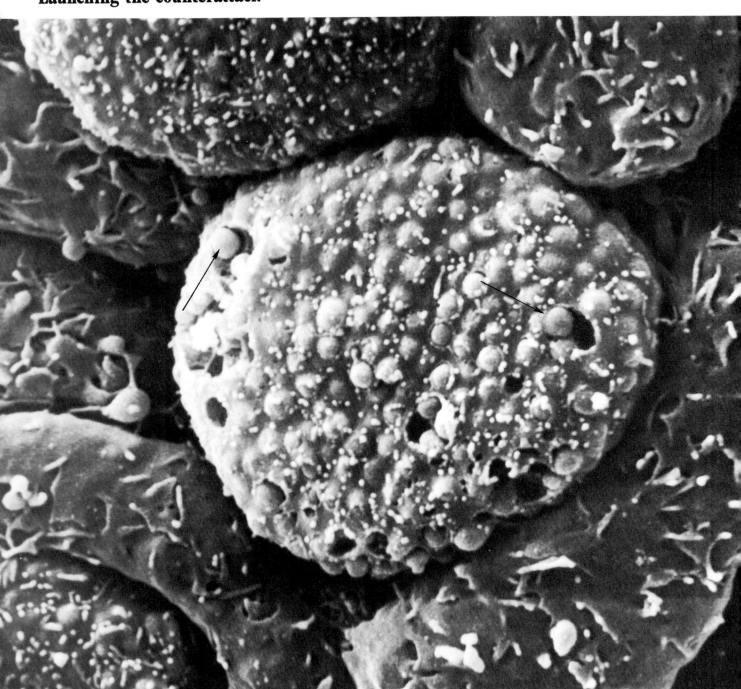

**INFLAMMATION—THE COLD SUFFERER'S FIRST CLUE**
*A specialized cell called a mast cell, magnified here about 8,000
times, emits granules (arrows) of histamine and other agents
that may contribute to inflammation—swelling, heat, redness and
pain in infected tissues. Inflammation helps produce sneezing
and coughing, which have a defensive effect.*

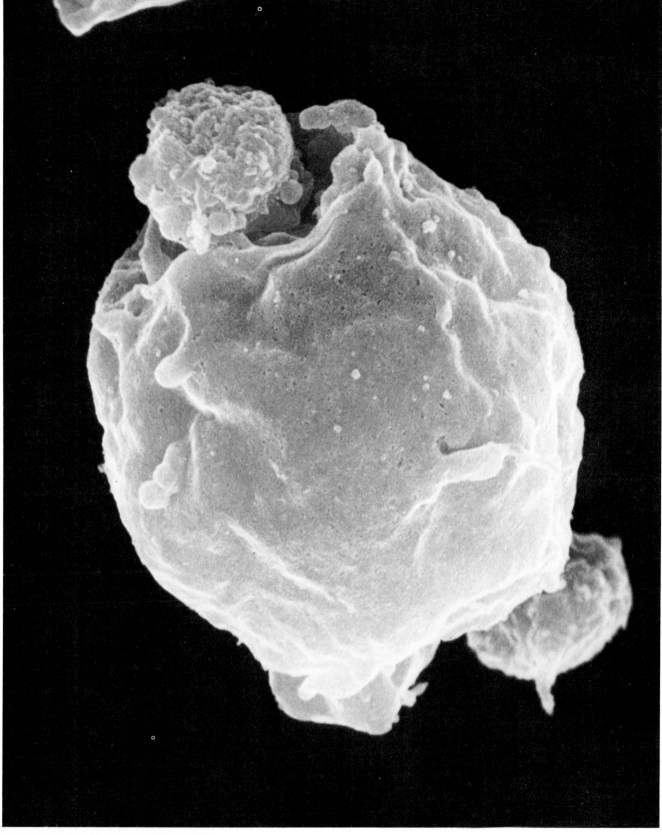

**ALL-PURPOSE SCAVENGING BY BIG EATERS**
*A macrophage, or big eater, engulfs a damaged cell (upper left). Big eaters are cells that clean up foreign or damaged material in the body; they function by consuming and digesting sick cells, viruses and bacteria, and become especially voracious when goaded by either infection or interferon.*

# The specialized virus fighters

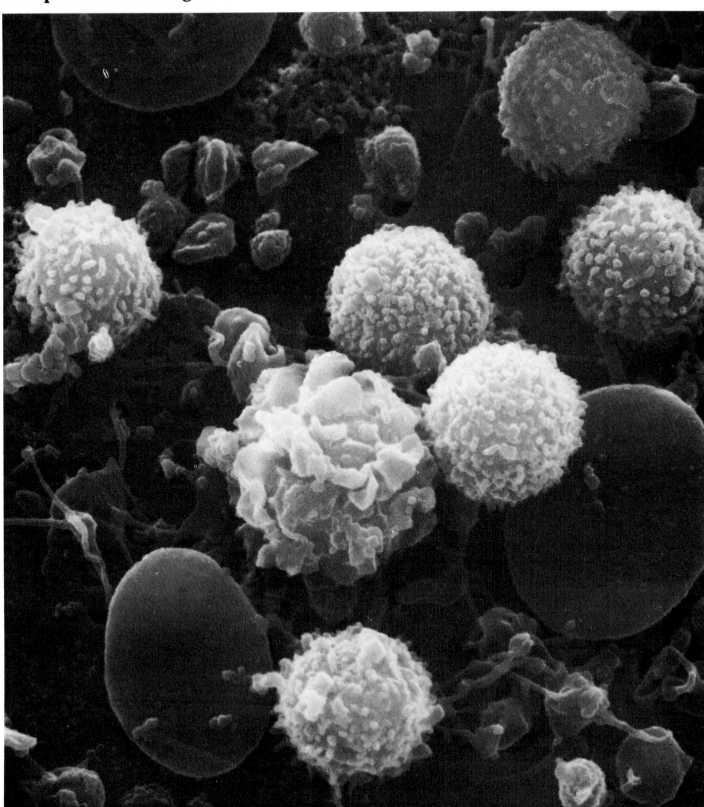

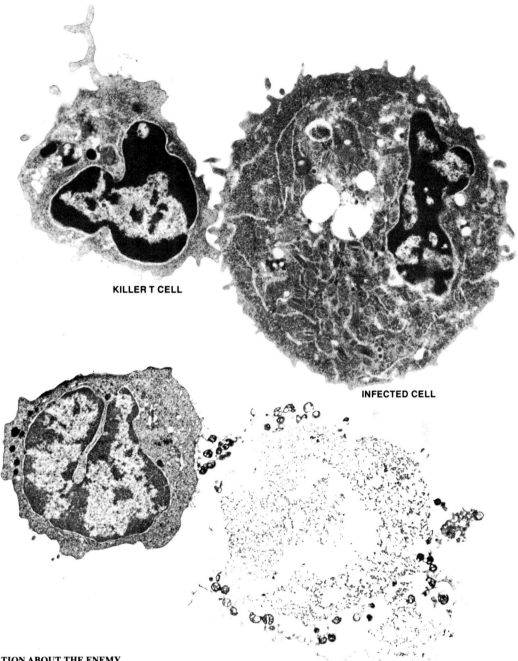

**KILLER T CELL**

**INFECTED CELL**

**AN EXCHANGE OF INFORMATION ABOUT THE ENEMY**
*Six bumpy-surfaced white blood cells—either T cells or B cells (pages 49 and 50)—approach a wrinkly big eater (center) that has ingested a virus-filled cell. The big eater presents the virus's unique markers for "reading" by the other cells, each of which can react only to a virus it matches. These specialized virus fighters then give off chemical signals that summon more defense cells from elsewhere in the body. The big dark forms are red blood cells; the smaller forms, blood platelets.*

**COUNTERATTACK BY A KILLER**
*The composite sequence above records the destruction of virus-laden mouse tissue by specialized white cells. At top a killer T cell releases corrosive proteins that will destroy a cell infected by a virus that the killer matches. At bottom, an attack has left only the ghostly remains of an infected cell. T-cell response peaks several days after cold symptoms appear.*

60

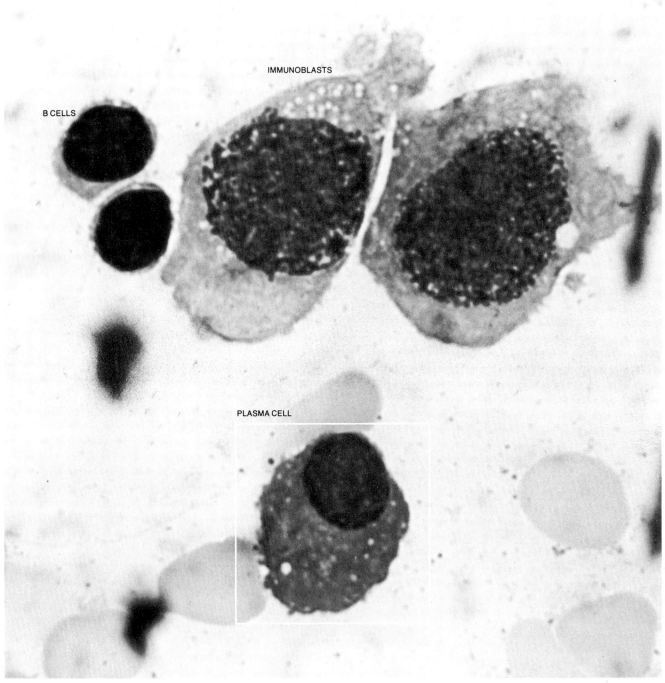

**MAKING ANTIBODIES TO STOP VIRUSES**
*This composite photomicrograph shows the three stages of*
*production of antibodies. Activated by contact with a virus they*
*match, specialized white cells called B cells change into a*
*larger cell called an immunoblast (upper sequence). At bottom, an*
*immunoblast becomes a plasma cell, which releases antibodies.*

**A FORM THAT BLOCKS VIRUS ACTIVITY**
*The antibodies produced by a plasma cell (below) block a virus by reacting chemically with its surface. The blocking effect is depicted below at right, with antibodies sketched as bow ties; viruses are pointed. The vulnerable cell is at right.*

**BLUNTING THE VIRUS KEY**
*When antibodies, which patrol the bloodstream for years after a virus has stimulated their production, meet that kind of virus, they cover the virus surface where it is keyed to match the vulnerable cell. In effect, the key on the virus surface—the point, in this illustration—is altered.*

**A CELL LOCKED AGAINST INVASION**
*After an antibody covers the key on the virus surface, the virus can no longer enter a vulnerable cell. The key—shown here as a point—no longer fits the corresponding area, shown as a notch, on the cell. Thus the virus cannot cause infection.*

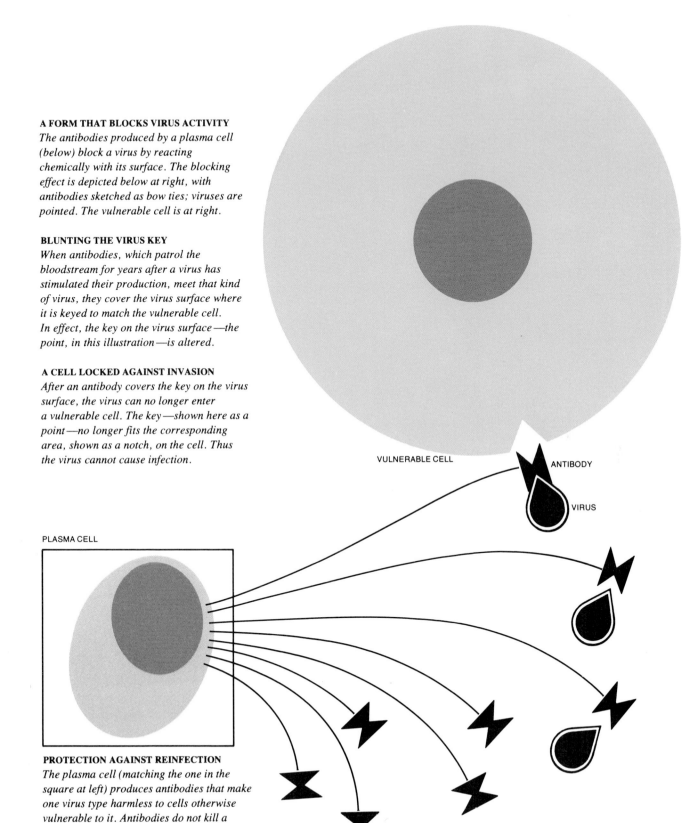

VULNERABLE CELL

ANTIBODY

VIRUS

PLASMA CELL

**PROTECTION AGAINST REINFECTION**
*The plasma cell (matching the one in the square at left) produces antibodies that make one virus type harmless to cells otherwise vulnerable to it. Antibodies do not kill a virus but prevent that type from reinfecting.*

# CHAPTER 3

# Treating the full-fledged cold

**Why there is no cure-all**
**What drugstore remedies can—and cannot—do**
**Relief for aches and sore muscles**
**Soothing a sore throat**
**A medicine chest for colds**

Whenever you sneeze, everyone within earshot is apt to respond with an earnest "God bless you." Your well-wishers might be surprised to learn that their casual expression of concern was once designed to ward off demons. The phrase goes back to ancient times, when the great explosion of air that accompanies a sneeze was widely believed to be caused by the soul leaving the body. Unless someone immediately spoke the protective words, demons would rush into the vacuum to take possession of the sneezer, and something far worse than a runny nose would surely follow.

As preventive medicine, "God bless you" has no known effect on the course of a cold. A good many other devices, however, do lessen the misery, if not the duration, of upper respiratory infection. The discomforts you experience during a cold—nasal blockage, headache, sneezing, sore throat, cough and, occasionally, hoarseness—are actually the secondary symptoms of a virtually unsensed viral invasion that your own body will eventually repel. If you can control, reduce or mask some of these symptoms, you can wait out the natural life of your cold in considerably better humor.

Dealing with the symptoms requires some understanding of them and of the treatments that are effective against them. At the first hint of what might be a cold, some people ransack the medicine cabinet to assemble a varied feast of remedies for any and all contingencies. This strategy is counterproductive on a number of scores. The cold—if that is what it is—has already taken up residence and cannot be nipped in the bud by any combination of drugs. Premature medication

will make it harder to evaluate the symptoms as they develop. And no drug, not even aspirin, is 100 per cent safe; when a disease is as mild as colds generally are, you and your body are best served by taking the least medication necessary.

Start your own cold regimen by making a few temporary changes in your normal patterns of behavior, and see if you do not feel a lot better right away. The first step is the simplest but, for many sufferers, the most difficult: Make up your mind to go easy on yourself for the next three or four days. If you feel lethargic or sleepy, get some extra rest; go to bed early or relax with a book until your energy returns. Stay home from work if your body tells you to. Your absence will not spare your associates—by the time your symptoms appear you have already exposed them to your viruses—but when you are demoralized and feel like a red-nosed pariah, you are probably not very efficient at whatever you do, and you will not accomplish much. Do not try to keep a cold-ridden child in bed during the day unless the youngster asks to go there, but do limit the child's activity.

If your appetite for solid food lags, do not be concerned; the old saw, Feed a cold and starve a fever, goes too far on both counts. Light, appealing, easily digested foods make nutritional sense for either a cold or a mild fever, but if all you feel like eating is lemon sherbet, give in to your whim. Comfort is the key issue; an eccentric diet during the few days that a cold lasts will have no lasting effect on your health.

Drink a lot of beverages. Fluids do not flush a cold away as was once believed, but they do work to loosen sticky mucus

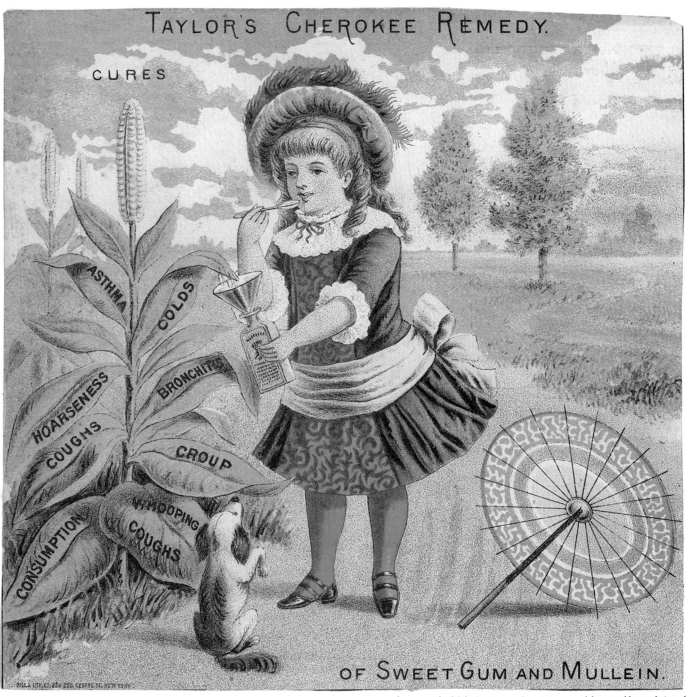

In an early-20th Century advertising card for a self-proclaimed cure-all for respiratory ailments, a girl performs an improbable chemical extraction from a mullein plant. The juice of mullein may suppress coughs, and sweet gum acts as an expectorant — but the most potent ingredient in this patent medicine was morphine, which stupefied the sufferer until the cold was gone.

in the upper respiratory passages, thus improving drainage and easing stuffiness. They also soothe a sore, dry throat and, in a body stricken by fever, replace water lost by increased perspiration. Unchilled fruit juices are good; their strong flavor gets through the most taste-deadening cold. Milk, which has a subtler flavor and a tendency to stimulate excess mucus flow in some people, may be among the least satisfactory fluids during a cold.

Alcoholic beverages are credited with semilegendary curative powers, and not by laymen alone: An old English medical text recommended that the patient "go home, hang his hat on the four poster, and proceed to drink whisky *quantum sufficit* to see two hats." This ancient pacifier has several drawbacks. Alcohol should never be mixed with any medicine you may take for a cold, because together they can add up to a dangerous dose of depressants. Even by itself, alcohol may add to existing nasal irritation, increasing congestion and headache while it temporarily diverts the drinker. If, after considering these facts, you still want a cocktail or a toddy, make it a weak one, then wait at least eight hours before taking any cold medication.

The best of all fluids for easing stuffiness are hot, non-alcoholic beverages. Researchers at Mt. Sinai Medical Center in Miami Beach, Florida, tested one time-honored miracle of medicine: hot chicken soup. Their experiment was a

model of objectivity and scientific precision. They first measured how long it took mucus to clear the nasal passages of a group that had taken no liquids for several hours. They then remeasured each person in the sample after administering identical doses of cold water, hot water and hot chicken soup.

The researchers found that the cold water decreased the speed at which mucus cleared the nasal passages by 2.8 millimeters per minute. Hot water speeded clearance by 2.2 millimeters, hot chicken soup by 2.3 millimeters. The fact that the subjects had inhaled water vapor while drinking the hot liquids accounted for the speed-up in clearance, and the soup may have won the contest by a nose: The researchers speculated that the aroma of the chicken in the broth somehow stimulated the nasal cilia to an extra tenth of a millimeter of effort. At best, the effects of the hot liquids were short-lived—normal nasal stuffiness returned in half an hour—but as chicken soup is nutritious, tasty and low in calories, there is no good reason not to follow Grandmother's advice. Drink the soup as often as you like. Hot tea and hot coffee are also beneficial beverages, but only in normal daily amounts.

Parents should monitor a child's intake of fluids with special care. Youngsters are more likely than adults to lose their appetite for liquids of any sort during a cold. If they refuse juice and water, try weak sweetened tea, soda pop that has been allowed to go flat, and warm soups or broths. A less familiar alternative is fruit-flavored gelatin desserts, in either jelled or liquid form, offered in small but frequent doses. Do not tempt a child with sweetened milk, milk shakes or ice cream, which may increase nasal secretion.

The next step beyond fluids taken by mouth is a home humidifier or vaporizer, but researchers are far from agreement on the value of either device for a run-of-the-mill cold. It was long believed that the dry, artificially heated indoor air of winter was a major contributor to the seasonal rise in colds, and many people equipped their homes and workplaces with large humidifying devices, generally as parts of heating and air-conditioning systems. But the importance of humidity in the spread of colds has been sharply downgraded, while the safety of the devices themselves has come into

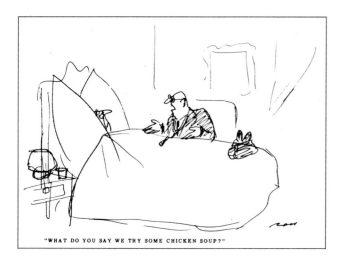

"WHAT DO YOU SAY WE TRY SOME CHICKEN SOUP?"

question. Cool-air humidifiers have been found to be breeding grounds for a variety of bacterial and fungal organisms that cause health problems of their own. If the water reservoir is not clean, a humidifier can broadcast agents that produce a reaction in some individuals, known as humidifier fever.

A different kind of humidifying device, the steam vaporizer sold in drugstores, has long been used to moisten the air around victims of respiratory diseases. Steam vaporizers are less likely to lead to infection because microorganisms cannot survive the heat of the steam, but bacteria and fungi can and do grow in the cooler plastic parts of these devices.

For some cold complications, such as the severe form of laryngitis called croup *(right),* a vaporizer is all but essential. With croup, increased humidity is the recommended treatment to ease labored breathing. The moisture in the air evaporates in the body's airways, cooling them and reducing the swelling of the larynx and lower airways that interferes with breathing. And if cough and nasal obstruction from an ordinary cold keep you from sleeping, a vaporizer on the floor of the bedroom may bring some relief.

Before plugging in a cool-mist machine, make sure that mineral deposits and slimy residues have been cleaned from the reservoir with a detergent since the device was last used; as long as you use the machine, change the water and clean the reservoir every day. Direct the flow of air so that it does not spray the cold sufferer directly but suffuses the room. You cannot, incidentally, improve a machine's effect on stuffiness by adding menthol, camphor, oil of eucalyptus or some other volatile substance to the water. Such substances may smell good but they have no proved therapeutic value, and they may cause additional irritation of the mucous membranes of the nose.

With or without the extra humidity, you will have to blow your nose now and then, and you will want to protect it from suffering any more abuse than it has to. There are in fact right ways and wrong ways to blow the nose. Avoid high-pressure blowing, or blowing one nostril at a time; instead, exhale gently through both nostrils, holding a handkerchief or tissue before the openings but touching and wiping the tender flesh as little as possible. The heroic honking some people pride

themselves on strains the blood vessels of the nose and strains the lungs; if the nasal passages are tightly obstructed, the pressure may backfire, forcing infected mucus deep into the sinuses or Eustachian tubes, where it can cause severe secondary complications.

For much the same reason, do not routinely sniff up runny material to clear your nose; if you have small children, take every opportunity before, during and after their colds to teach

## Coping with croup

Few ailments of early childhood are more frightening to parents than the severe form of laryngitis called croup. Occurring mainly in children under three, croup usually begins with an ordinary cold. Then suddenly—often in the middle of the night—the child awakens, gasping for air. The characteristic symptom is a high-pitched cough, similar to a seal's bark—an indication that airways to the lungs are partially closed by spasms, swelling and thick secretions of mucus.

Although croup seems to threaten asphyxiation, it is rarely serious. The choking cough can generally be relieved by humid air. A cold-mist vaporizer is helpful: The mist will thin the secretions and reduce the swelling. Sitting with a croup-stricken child in a bathroom made steamy by a hot shower also works. If breathing difficulties persist after 20 minutes of treatment with mist or steam, call a physician or take the child to a hospital.

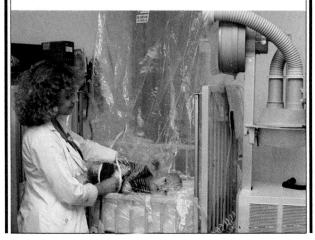

*Comforted by a nurse, a small child is treated for croup at Children's Hospital in San Diego, California. The patient lies in a portable, transparent tent, in which the air is filled with a cool mist. Cool moist air is preferable to steam because it will not aggravate a fever, but they are equally effective.*

them how to blow their noses, so that they will not develop the sniffling habit. Very young children often have a difficult time with nasal obstruction. Feeding periods are particularly troublesome: It is all but impossible to suck from a bottle or nurse at the breast while breathing through the mouth. You can improve a child's labored breathing by using an infant nasal aspirator, a rubber bulb fitted with a plastic siphon, to draw off accumulated mucus and clear the nasal passages just before the child's feeding time.

Less troublesome than stuffiness, but often just as irritating, is what might be called the red-nose syndrome, which almost everyone suffers at some stage of a cold. To reduce this unpleasant result of chapping and frequent wiping, daub

a little petroleum jelly on the affected area. The treatment works particularly well if you apply the jelly just before going to sleep, so that it will be undisturbed for several hours.

**Why there is no cure-all**

Now that you have made a few concessions to your cold, have put your feet up and downed a few cups of juice and soup, you may feel good enough to wait out the next seven days. But suppose you still feel awful, or suppose you must get on with your life and cannot afford to sit back while the cold goes away. Two possibilities are open to you. You can seek relief from one or more of the cough and cold medicines fervently described in magazine and TV advertisements. Or,

## Safety precautions for vaporizers and humidifiers

The most pleasant sound a cold sufferer can hear may be the gentle whoosh or whir of a gadget that adds moisture to the air. The extra humidity eases breathing by loosening mucus that can block respiratory passages. Two plug-in appliances, the vaporizer and the humidifier, work differently but produce the same result. Both require special precautions for safe operation.

The moist, cool interior of a humidifier, which sprays mist into

the air from a spinning disk, is a fertile breeding ground for mildew and disease-spreading microorganisms. Clean and wipe the water reservoir every day, and disinfect internal parts every five days. A vaporizer humidifies the air by generating steam when a pair of electrodes passes electricity through water. The possibility of spilling scalding water is obviously a hazard; keep a vaporizer away from exposed locations or areas used by children.

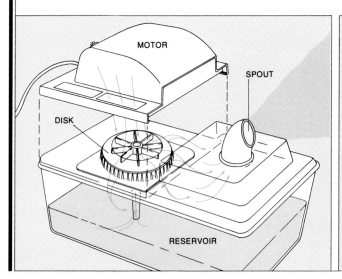

**ANATOMY OF A HUMIDIFIER**
*The motor of this typical humidifier spins a finned disk that mixes water and air in a fine mist and drives it out through a spout. To disinfect the unit, fill the reservoir halfway with water and add a half cup of liquid laundry bleach. Plug the spout with a cloth, run the motor 90 minutes, then wash all parts with soapy water.*

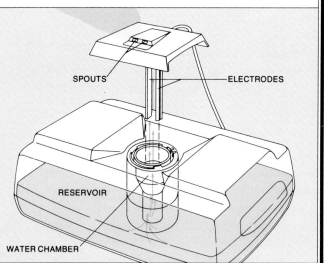

**ANATOMY OF A VAPORIZER**
*Within the reservoir of this vaporizer, electrodes feed electricity into a small water chamber, generating enough heat to boil the water. The resulting steam condenses as it leaves the spouts, humidifying the air. After two days' operation, scrape mineral deposits from the disconnected electrodes with a screwdriver.*

more drastically, you can go to your family doctor for an elixir dispensed only by prescription.

The second possibility is the easier to dispose of: Save yourself time and money by not calling your doctor. If your cold is nothing more than a cold, if your temperature is no higher than 102° F. (38° C.) and if you have no chronic ailments that might be aggravated by an upper respiratory infection, there is nothing a doctor can do for you that you cannot do as well or better for yourself. Prescription cold preparations are similar to the nonprescription formulas you can buy at a pharmacy; antibiotics such as penicillin, tetracycline and erythromycin, which are also sold by prescription, can work miracles against bacterial infections but are useless in fighting the common cold or any other viral infection.

The explanation for antibiotics' unfortunate limitations lies in the different physical natures of bacteria and viruses. Bacteria exist as separate living organisms, independent of human cells. Their complex metabolic and reproductive processes, upon which their survival depends, are vulnerable to the action of antibiotics; when an antibiotic and bacteria come into contact, the antibiotic disrupts the bacteria's life cycle, ending further infection. Viruses, by contrast, exist within their host's cells and become part of the host cell structure, out of reach of any antimicrobial substance.

Some doctors will prescribe an antibiotic for a patient who demands it, on the theory that even if it does not do any direct good, it will at least not do any harm. Experience has shown, however, that the casual use of antibiotics can do very serious harm indeed. In *Current Therapy,* a standard desk reference for physicians, Dr. C. Alan Phillips of the University of Vermont College of Medicine summed up the dangers of using antibiotics against an acute viral infection. They have no antiviral action, and they may encourage the emergence of resistant organisms. In addition, serious toxic or allergic reactions to these potent drugs may occur. The patient may be sensitized to the antibacterial drug and thus be denied the use of an important therapeutic agent during a subsequent serious bacterial infection.

For these reasons, do not ask a doctor for an antibiotic unless there is a clear indication that a respiratory infection has bacterial complications. And be firm in turning down antibiotics proffered by a well-meaning friend. Too often, someone will try to present you with some leftover antibiotic pills or capsules that "cleared up a cold overnight." You can be sure that the friend's vanquished cold was not a cold or that the antibiotic was irrelevant to the recovery. It will certainly be irrelevant to the course of your own cold and may prove detrimental to your health.

**What drugstore remedies can—and cannot—do**

With no antiviral medicine yet available, the best drug treatment is medicine you can buy without a prescription, over the counter, or OTC, in pharmacists' jargon. There are hundreds designed to alleviate the symptoms of a cold. Most work, after a fashion. And most are safe, more or less. But to a great extent, buyers of cold remedies are on their own in evaluating the safety and effectiveness of over-the-counter drugs.

Governments are traditionally reluctant to regulate the medical business, and only recently have scientists come to understand the actions of many of these drugs on the body's mechanisms. Even in the United States, for example, where medicines are strictly regulated, the chief regulatory agency in the field of drugs, the Food and Drug Administration (FDA), used to limit its responsibility to the monitoring of drugs for toxicity alone. Claims of effectiveness were left largely to the discretion of drug manufacturers—whose opinion of their own products was, not surprisingly, often generous in the extreme. By the same token, drug manufacturers were not regulated closely in the combinations of approved agents they chose to put together. The FDA raised no objections, for example, to the inclusion of infinitesimal quantities of antihistamines, even when those agents were irrelevant to the symptoms allegedly being treated or were present in amounts too small to be effective.

In 1972, however, at the FDA's request, 17 professional panels, composed of nongovernment experts, including health care professionals, drug specialists, representatives from the OTC drug industry, and consumers, reviewed OTC products for effectiveness, safety, labeling and advertising claims. The cold and cough remedies panel considered

# Deadly complications from bacteria

Colds and influenza, being mild viral infections of the respiratory tract, pose no serious threat to health. Yet cold and flu victims are routinely warned to be alert for symptoms that exceed the usual ones. Though the original infection may not be dangerous, complications that can follow it may be deadly. The most alarming secondary infection is also caused by a virus *(page 116),* but some serious complications arise from bacteria, which are totally different from viruses.

Four types of bacteria cause the majority of cold and flu complications. One type, staphylococcus, can infect the lungs, to produce a particularly severe form of pneumonia, most often in infants and elderly people. Another type, called pneumococcus, causes a more common pneumonia that annually strikes 500,000 people and kills 25,000 in the United States alone. Pneumococcus can also produce middle-ear and sinus infections. A third type, *Hemophilus influenzae,* also attacks the middle ear and the sinuses, and the infection may recur again and again for months.

The fourth type of dangerous bacterial agent is Group A streptococcus *(below).* It, too, can cause pneumonia, although it rarely does so. It can also infect the tonsils or middle ear, but it is best known for the painful and potentially deadly strep throat, which often sweeps through crowded communities such as schools,

camps and military training centers. Children are particularly susceptible; according to one estimate, as many as 20 per cent of all school children suffer at least one bout of strep throat every year. Left untreated, this ailment can lead to kidney disease, rheumatic fever or other life-threatening illness.

When these dangers arise, it is not simply because colds and flu make the body easier for bacteria to invade. An invasion may not be necessary—often, the bacteria are already in the body, sharing living space with a vast variety of bacteria that are innocuous or even beneficial to human life. The potential destroyers generally do nothing to upset good health. But when a cold or flu wears down the body's defenses, and congestion-blocked passageways collect pockets of mucus that serve as incubators, the harmful germs multiply and spread. They then generate a second, bacterial illness on top of the first, viral illness.

Fortunately, bacterial infections, unlike most viral diseases, are treatable. Bacteria are much larger than viruses—the streptococcus pictured is more than 30 times the size of the most common cold virus—and are complete living organisms rather than the simple packet of hereditary material forming a virus. Bacteria can be killed by antibiotics, if the drugs are administered in time—hence the need for alertness to unusual symptoms.

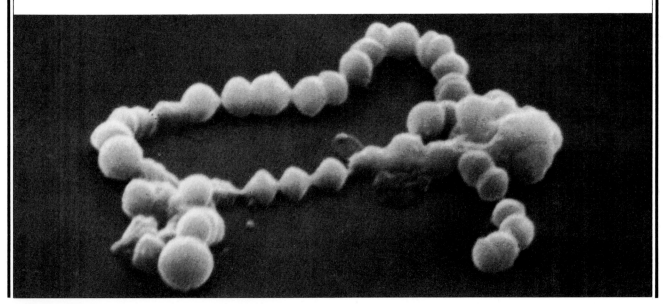

*A string of Group A streptococcus bacteria, magnified 16,000 times by a scanning electron microscope, looks somewhat like a necklace of harmless pearls. In fact, these bacteria are a serious source of secondary illness, including sore throat, tonsillitis, middle-ear infection and pneumonia.*

some 50,000 products containing over 120 active ingredients. Its judgments, backed by new scientific knowledge of drug actions and effects, reinforced doubts about the value of many cold remedies.

The panel found that the makers of so-called shotgun remedies, which combine many drugs in a single preparation, often load the mixture with agents that the user may not need. An individual cold might require no more than a decongestant, or a painkiller, or a cough suppressant—but the consumer often gets all three, and possibly other substances for good measure. One understandably popular cold remedy is 25 per cent alcohol, which makes it the equivalent of 50-proof liquor. The panel recommended that manufacturers produce more single-agent products, targeted at single symptoms, so that cold sufferers could custom tailor a drug program to the specific symptoms that cause discomfort. Predictably, the panel also called for improvements in labeling and advertising, which it found generally "overly complicated, vague, unsupported by scientific evidence, and in some cases, misleading."

Until recommendations like these take wide effect, you can expect to find a good many useless, even counterproductive, drugs mixed in with the worthwhile cough and cold medicines on your pharmacist's shelves. To make informed choices, you will need to know something about the most common agents found in cold preparations—what symptoms, if any, each treats, and what its drawbacks may be.

Even the form in which the drug is compounded—tablets, capsules, liquid, spray or jelly—is a consideration. Some cold pills are timed-release tablets, many containing combinations of several drugs. Designed to release small doses over a period of several hours, the timed-release products work well as bedtime medicines, giving modest but sustained relief through the night. In the daytime, when rapid relief is what is wanted, their delayed action may make them less desirable than similar drugs in more conventional forms.

The best place to start your short course in self-medication is in the labels on cough and cold products. Though the language there may seem foreign or arcane, you can easily decipher it, and virtually everything you need to know is available. Here are some items of information that American and some European manufacturers provide, though not necessarily in this order:

● The registered name of a patent medicine and a category in which a medicine may be classed, such as decongestant, nasal spray or aspirin. Use this item to tell the kind of product you are buying as well as its better-known trade name.

● The symptom or symptoms the product is alleged to relieve. Though manufacturers' claims are not always reliable, this item can help you choose a product that acts on the symptoms you have rather than those you are free of.

● An expiration date for drugs that have a limited shelf life. By law, all over-the-counter drugs that lose their effectiveness over a period of time must have an expiration date stamped on the label. (Products that do not have a limited shelf life, such as cough drops and rubbing alcohol, are not affected by the law and do not bear an expiration date.) Do not use any drug after its expiration date.

● The chemical names and quantities per tablet or spoonful of the active ingredients—that is, the chemical substances that do the actual work of the medicine. Measurements are given in metric units: milligrams, or mg., for tablets; cubic centimeters, or cc., for liquids. An exception is some brands of aspirin or aspirin substitutes, which in the United States may be measured by the grain, or gr., a traditional apothecaries' unit equal to 64.8 milligrams. Nontherapeutic binders such as salt, sugar and water need not be listed but often are. Use this item to choose the safest, most effective ingredients, as described in the next section of this chapter. Use it, too, if you are sensitive or allergic to specific ingredients, and do not ignore the nontherapeutic ingredients if they are listed. For example, many medications contain large amounts of nontherapeutic sodium—a fact of great importance to anyone suffering from heart disease, high blood pressure or any other condition calling for a sodium-restricted diet.

● Directions for use, including the method of taking the medication (chewing, swallowing, spraying and so forth) and the recommended dosages. Follow these directions exactly; never overdose and, if special directions are given for children, never treat a child with an adult dosage. Use this item, too, to help determine whether the quantity you buy will be sufficient for the probable duration of the illness.

● Warnings, including the maximum daily dosage, the limit on the duration of continuous treatment, possible adverse side effects, and circumstances that require a doctor's supervision in taking the medicine, such as a history of diabetes or high blood pressure. The label also includes any appropriate precautions against adverse interactions with other drugs the user may be taking. Read all of this information with special care: No drug, remember, is completely safe. Because cold medicines at best relieve symptoms without curing the infection, you may well want to weigh the risks of taking them against the temporary benefits they bring.

## Six basic types of active ingredients

Of all the items on a label, perhaps the most important to a cold sufferer are the active ingredients—they are, after all, the reason the remedy was purchased in the first place. Over-the-counter preparations typically contain active agents that purport to treat from one to six different categories of symptoms. These agents are:

● Anticholinergics, to temporarily relieve watery secretions in the nose and eyes.

● Nasal decongestants, to clear the nasal passages.

● Antihistamines, to relieve sneezing and runny nose.

● Antitussives, to suppress coughs.

● Expectorants, to thin and loosen accumulated mucus in the airways of the respiratory tract.

● Painkillers, or analgesics, to reduce fever and soothe aches and pains.

The cold and cough remedies panel found some of these agents truly helpful, others of no use at all.

Anticholinergics are used in conjunction with other agents in combination cold products. They were found by the panel to be of no therapeutic value. The most common form, atropine or a mixture of belladonna alkaloids, is restricted to levels of .2 milligram or less in OTC products because of risks associated with higher concentrations: Neither showed any evidence of reducing secretions due to colds. The American Pharmaceutical Association, a professional pharmacists'

organization, concurred with this judgment, and added that an individual hypersensitive to atropine or suffering from asthma, glaucoma or enlarged prostate should not take anticholinergics, even in small quantities, without consulting a physician. Other people should choose the recipe with the smallest amount of anticholinergic indicated on the label, all other therapeutic features being comparable.

Nasal decongestants produce a stimulating effect on the nervous system that causes small blood vessels to constrict. In a cold victim, they act on swollen blood vessels in the mucus-secreting areas of the nose, causing the vessels to shrink to normal size. The constriction results in reduced blood flow, reduced fluid in surrounding tissues and more open space in the nasal passages. Breathing may become easier, drainage of the nose and sinuses may return to normal, and pain due to irritation of nerve endings in the nose may diminish as pressure is relieved.

The decongestants used in over-the-counter products are made up in several forms: sprays, jellies and nose drops, all of which are applied to a specific surface area and affect only that area; and oral drugs, such as pills, which are absorbed by the entire body. The forms differ chiefly in their duration of action and in the hazards they present to persons with such chronic conditions as hyperthyroidism, heart disease, high blood pressure and diabetes, which are aggravated by any constriction of blood vessels.

The topical decongestants—those applied directly to the suffering area—generally produce more dramatic, quick-acting effects in clearing the nose. However, in many cases, partial stuffiness quickly returns, and some people then ignore the label directions, either repeating the application sooner than directed or using doses larger than the recommended amounts. Either practice can lead to local irritation and to a rebound effect, in which the active ingredient reduces congestion, as it is meant to do, but at the same time stimulates more congestion. The rebound syndrome is so common that pharmacists call it by an impressive name: *rhinitis medicamentosa*. Severe *rhinitis medicamentosa* may end in permanent damage to the nasal membranes.

Topical decongestants also have drawbacks arising from

# The motley potions and gadgets of yesteryear

When great-grandfather went out to buy something for his cold, he found choices far richer—if not better—than those of today. Many of the examples below and on the following pages, from the Smithsonian Institution, remain useful in modern form. Others were shorter-lived for a variety of reasons.

Some, such as cough medicines laced with opiates, were effec-

tive but very dangerous. A number reflect medical beliefs that no longer are popular. But most were doomed by overzealous claims. Typical was the boast of Dr. R. V. Pierce that a cold victim who tried Dr. Pierce's Golden Medical Discovery (*below, top left*) "finds his whole person has been entirely renovated and repaired, he feels like a new man—a perfect being."

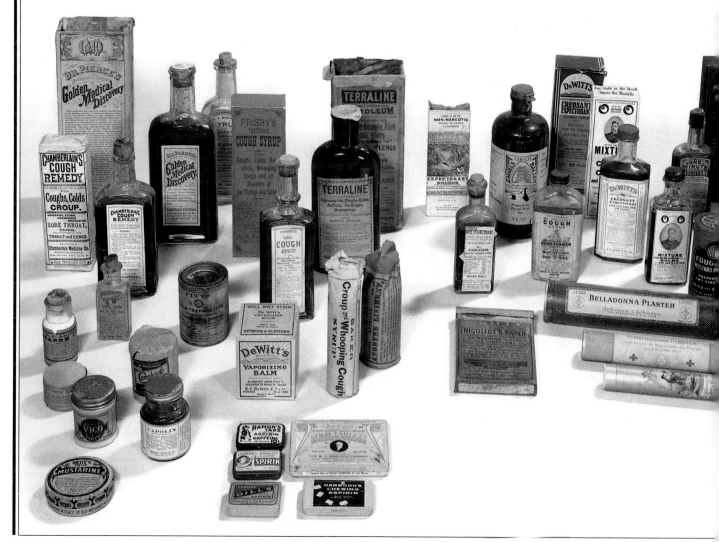

*Almost all of the labels on this panoply of turn-of-the-century patent medicines, including cough syrups (rear), salves (lower left), pills (center) and plasters (right), touted an "immediate and permanent cure" for every respiratory disease known.*

*A decongestant called Cresolene (right) was sold with its own vaporizer (center). The saucer was filled with Cresolene and the oil burner in the base was lighted, sending fumes throughout the room.*

*When the water inside this elaborate vaporizer was boiled by the alcohol burner, the cold sufferer breathed the vapor from the glass funnel and thus humidified his respiratory tract to relieve stuffiness.*

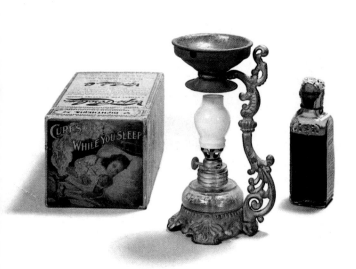

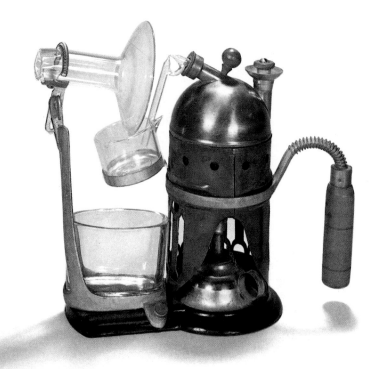

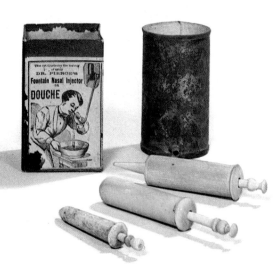

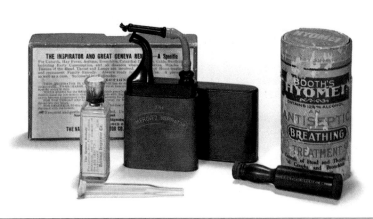

*Nose rinses were popular 19th Century treatments. The Nasal Douche was filled with medicine and operated as shown on the box. The three syringes were used to squeeze ointment into nose and ears.*

*Inhalants from these flasks were to clear stuffy noses. The Improved Inspirator has breathing attachments for both mouth (left) and nose, and a metal cover. Hyomei was inhaled directly from its black bottle.*

The bright-red Lung Protector was simply a felt vest for a child. More effective at countering a cold's chills were metal hot-water bottles—the one at top has an indentation to keep a cup of broth warm.

Dr. Fuller's Electro Spiral Magnetic Vegetable Vapor Cure is nothing more than a bottle with a sponge wedged into the top and bottom and soaked with a "vegetable compound," to be inhaled.

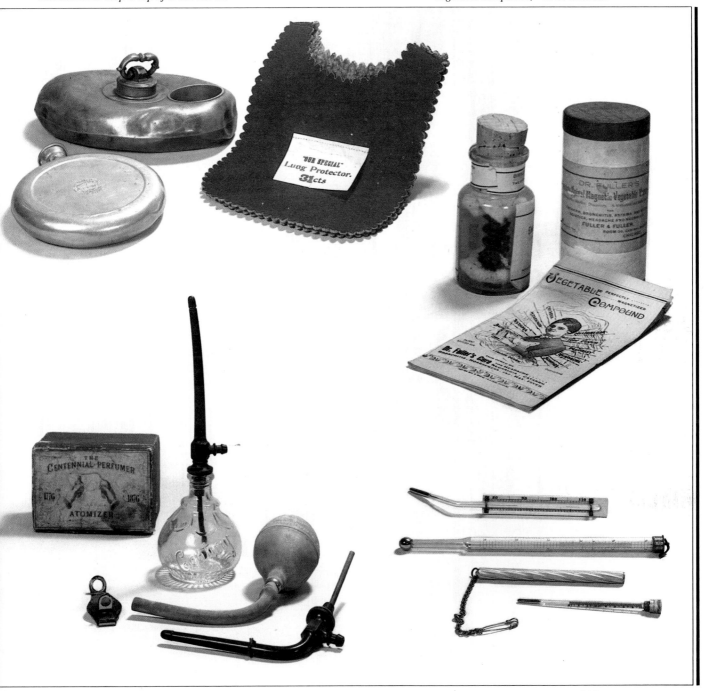

The Century Atomizer sprayed mist into the nose when the rubber bulb, affixed to the side of the dispensing attachment, was squeezed. The attachment in the foreground was used to spray the throat.

The most unusual of these three old fever thermometers is the dog-legged one at top. The thermometer at bottom screws into its spiral case and probably was used by a nurse and pinned to her uniform.

the ways they are administered. Aerated sprays do not deliver a standard dose with each squeeze of the bottle: Pressure on a nearly full container produces more spray than the same pressure on a nearly empty one. And as anyone who has had a very stuffy nose will remember, getting a spray to penetrate deep into the nose can be as difficult as getting a breeze to pass through a closed window. Drops, on the other hand, can be measured with reasonable accuracy and usually do a good job of getting through impacted mucus, but they do not spread themselves as effectively as spray. If the medication is not administered correctly, a substantial portion will end up in the throat and be swallowed without having done its job. And while nose drops are safe for topical application, they can cause problems once they are absorbed. The third type of topical decongestant, jelly, is applied just inside the nose. It may be less effective than the others, because it does not get far enough inside the nose to reach the inflamed area.

For maximum effectiveness from a topical decongestant, observe the following procedures. First, gently blow your nose to clear it of any excess mucus. If you are using a spray,

## A mislabeled ailment's hidden dangers

Cold sores or fever blisters—the familiar small blisters that erupt around the edges of the lips—are badly misnamed. They are not caused by either colds or fever; they are symptoms of an infection by a virus, herpes simplex type 1, that has fascinated scientists for decades.

Most people contract herpes in childhood, often without showing any symptoms at all. Normally, the body's defenses bring the virus under control within two weeks, but they do not kill it outright and they do not confer immunity against subsequent infections: Virologists believe that the herpes virus takes up permanent residence in nerves around the mouth. Some herpes victims are never bothered again, but most of them suffer occasional cold sores, when the virus migrates from the nerves and infects the skin; in the United States alone, at least 50 million people undergo one or more outbreaks of cold sores every year. These episodes can be triggered by any physical or psychological stress—not only colds and fever, but acute anxiety, menstruation, and skin irritation from shaving, kissing or sunburn.

The blisters that signal the start of an attack generally rupture about four days after they first appear; the yellow, crusted scabs they leave behind heal without scarring in about a week. In themselves, both the sores and the scabs are harmless, though they are always irritating and sometimes rather painful. The only treatment needed is an antibiotic ointment, which reduces painful cracking of the skin and prevents bacteria from invading the sore. Current research, however, holds promise of both a preventive vaccine and a cure for recurrent infection.

The real hazard of herpes infections is that a victim's saliva and blister fluid contain live virus, which can invade any microscopic skin abrasion. Herpes simplex type 1 also can infect the genital organs, although venereal infections caused by a different virus, herpes simplex type 2, are more common. Worst of all, the type 1 virus can cause eye infections that damage the cornea—the transparent tissue forming the outer coat of the eyeball—and the resulting scars are the second leading cause of blindness in the United States.

The virus spreads only in saliva or by direct physical contact—unlike cold viruses, herpes virus is rapidly inactivated once outside living cells—but transmission is easy. Herpes victims frequently unwittingly give themselves secondary infections: A thumb-sucker, for example, can infect a cut thumb; others may scratch a sore, then rub their eyes or handle contact lenses. The virus can be spread from one person to another by a shared drinking glass or by kissing—even a soothing kiss to a child's cut or burn can transmit an infection. Some occupations or activities are peculiarly prone to infection; dentists, for example, frequently contract herpes infections on their fingers from their patients' saliva, and wrestlers suffer skin infections when the virus invades a superficial abrasion.

Herpes carriers cannot entirely control the spread of the disease, because their saliva may contain live virus even when they do not have a sore. But when blisters appear, they can minimize the risk by washing their hands frequently, avoiding kissing and resisting the temptation to scratch a sore or rub their eyes. Such precautions are particularly important when the blisters first form, because the fluid they contain is laden with live virus. After about five days, when the blister sites are encrusted with scabs, cold sores are no longer contagious.

hold your head upright and insert the tip of the sprayer into a nostril, then squeeze the center of the container once and sniff in at the same time. Repeat the process in each nostril for the recommended number of times, return the cap to the applicator and tighten it, and sniff in two or three times more, drawing the contents of the spray deep into the nasal passages. If possible, avoid touching any part of your nose with the sprayer tip. Some viruses and bacteria are bound to lodge on the tip; therefore do not share a container with anyone else, and throw it away when the cold is over.

If you are using nose drops, find a comfortable position in which you can tilt your head way back; lying on a bed with your head over the edge is generally the best arrangement. Apply the recommended number of drops to each nostril and remain in position for five minutes, breathing through your mouth and rotating your head gently to spread the medication. Because the applicator usually becomes contaminated, dispose of the drops when the cold ends.

Pills generally give longer-lasting action than the topical medications and are seldom associated with rebound effects. On the negative side, they give somewhat less relief, because they do not produce the same high degree of blood vessel constriction and they act more slowly. Absorbed into the body's entire system, they also excite the nervous system sufficiently to cause insomnia in some persons if taken just before bedtime—and to worsen the excess stimulation that afflicts those who have an overactive thyroid gland. Because pills constrict all blood vessels, not just those in the nose, they should be avoided by persons with heart disease and high blood pressure. Decongestants may also worsen diabetes; they increase the sugar in the blood, intensifying the harm caused by the diabetic's own bodily malfunction. Anyone on some other course of drug therapy—especially persons taking monoamine oxidase inhibitor, often prescribed for depression—should consult a physician before taking decongestant pills, which interact with many other drugs.

Among the entire array of decongestants, most people find that spray, though slightly more expensive, is more convenient than drops or jelly, and probably more effective than oral types. Spray is also generally preferable for children who are old enough to sniff in the decongestant and blow their noses between applications; for infants and toddlers drops are better, but should be formulated especially for children. Oral decongestants are recommended mainly for adults whose congestion discomfort extends to the chest or who have experienced problems with topical decongestants; their general health must, of course, permit use of these whole-body drugs. No topical decongestant should be used for more than three to four days and no oral decongestant for more than seven days without a doctor's recommendation.

In any form—pills, jellies, drops or spray—one of the most effective and popular decongestant compounds is phenylephrine. Naphazoline is more potent than phenylephrine, and more likely to cause irritation; it is, therefore, usually made up in drop form, but even drops may produce a slight stinging sensation when first applied. Deongestant drops containing naphazoline should not be given to children. Ephedrine, a derivative of a plant of the Ephedra genus, is the topical decongestant in longest use, and indeed was used in ancient China for relief of congestion and asthma. It can be administered in oily solutions, but the FDA panel approved only water-based solutions; the oil-based products present some risk of complications leading to a form of pneumonia.

Levodesoxyephedrine and propylhexedrine are two similar agents commonly used in sprays. They can irritate the nose and may slow the action of nasal cilia. Oxymetazoline and xylometazoline are longer acting than the other topical decongestants mentioned—the recommended dose is given only twice a day, with maximum relief lasting up to six hours and diminished relief continuing for another six hours.

The decongestant drugs most frequently made up as pills include ephedrine, phenylpropanolamine and pseudoephedrine. In oral form, ephedrine stimulates the nervous system, and several preparations include a depressant, which overcomes this side effect. Ephedrine's relief begins within an hour of swallowing a pill and lasts from three to four hours. The other two agents peak later, last longer and leave little nervous stimulation in their train.

The third class of drugs found in over-the-counter medicines is antihistamines. In the view of the review panel, their

## Codeine — a grand old cough remedy

Few cures have come down from the days of medicine shows and snake oil with their respectability intact. One that has, and that remains the most effective treatment available for the malady it alleviates, is codeine—the opium derivative that has been a sovereign remedy for coughs since shortly after it was first isolated as an impurity of morphine by the French pharmacist Pierre-Jean Robiquet in 1832.

Codeine, like other opiates, suppresses the urge to cough by desensitizing the part of the brain that triggers the muscles of the coughing mechanism. In heavy doses it also induces sleep, a side effect that can be helpful to a cold or flu victim, since rest speeds recovery from the virus infection. However, like many opiates, codeine can, after continued consumption, so alter body chemistry that the user becomes an addict, suffering withdrawal symptoms if denied regular doses.

In the 19th and early 20th Centuries, codeine was freely dispensed in high concentrations—not only to suppress coughs but also to relieve pain and combat diarrhea (both of which it does effectively). Some users became addicted without even knowing they were taking a narcotic. Because of this danger the sale of codeine has come under stringent legal control, particularly in the United States.

Federal law classifies codeine preparations into several categories of availability, depending on the concentration of the drug. The most effective cough suppressants, containing 1.8 or more per cent codeine, require a written one-time-only prescription. Medicines with less than 1.8 but more than .2 per cent of the drug may be prescribed by telephone and refilled, and those with still less may be dispensed by a pharmacist without a prescription but with the sales recorded in a register. Even stricter controls have been applied by a number of states, and some prohibit the sale of any codeine-containing medicine without a prescription.

Because of the legal restrictions on codeine, most of the nonprescription cough medicines sold in America contain no codeine at all. Of 112 brands examined in 1977, all but one were combinations of expectorant, decongestant, antihistamine, soothing compound, antiseptic, local anesthetic and cough suppressant. In most brands the suppressant was dextromethorphan, a synthetic considered nonaddictive. Its power to suppress coughs is virtually equal to that of the legal amount of codeine in nonprescription remedies.

value in relieving cold symptoms is unproved, yet they continue to turn up as an ingredient in many broad-range cold brews. Antihistamines probably found their niche in these medicines because they do relieve the seasonal coldlike symptoms of allergies such as hay fever, characterized by a runny nose, itching eyes, sneezing and swollen nasal tissue.

In allergies, antihistamines diminish these unpleasant symptoms by acting against a natural body substance called histamine, which causes them. Histamine is normally stored in the body, but it is released when certain cells are stimulated by allergic agents such as pollen. Once out of storage and in circulation, histamine causes the dilation of blood vessels, the seepage of fluid into surrounding tissue spaces and a runny nose. A viral invasion of the nose will also cause the release of histamine, but in this case the quantity of histamine in circulation has relatively minor significance. The body's response to the virus alone—that is, the appearance of a full-fledged cold—is fully capable of bringing on all the same symptoms without the release of histamine, and taking antihistamines is essentially an exercise in futility.

Besides their dubious value in treating colds, antihistamines create problems that often make their presence in cold preparations, even in small amounts, undesirable. They cause drowsiness, and are dangerous to use before driving, working with machinery or engaging in any other activity that requires full attention and energy. Because they greatly enhance the soporific effects of other substances, they should not be combined with alcohol, sleeping pills, tranquilizers or painkillers. In people suffering from glaucoma, antihistamines can raise pressure—within the eye or the arteries—and complicate treatment.

Men suffering from an enlarged prostate gland should also be cautious with antihistamines; they restrict the elimination of urine, intensifying the urination difficulty caused by the prostate ailment. And a physician's supervision is advisable in antihistamine treatment of children with convulsive disorders: Although these drugs ordinarily cause drowsiness, they paradoxically can stimulate children; in those already afflicted by overstimulated nervous systems, the illness may be worsened. Pregnant women and nursing mothers should avoid cold preparations that contain even small amounts of antihistamine because the ingested drug may have undesirable effects on the developing fetus or the infant.

The next two classes of chemical agents—the antitussives, or cough suppressants, and the expectorants—are taken sometimes separately, sometimes together, depending on the type of cough involved. In what is known as a nonproductive cough, the muscular reflex of coughing is constantly stimulated by inflammation in the throat, but little mucus is produced or ejected. A productive cough, on the other hand, brings up quantities of mucus and contributes to their removal. The objective of an antitussive is to silence a nonproductive cough; that of an expectorant, to enhance the effectiveness of a productive cough without increasing its frequency.

Cough suppressants include both narcotic and nonnarcotic agents that lull the cough control center in the brain so that it triggers the cough reflex less often. The most effective is the narcotic codeine, a derivative of opium. Because its use can lead to addiction, the amount of codeine in over-the-counter cold remedies is strictly controlled in the United States.

Codeine does not affect the cough mechanism alone. It occasionally produces nausea, drowsiness, allergic reactions and constipation (it is, in fact, used as an antidiarrhea drug). Over-the-counter cough suppressants containing codeine should not be taken, without a physician's approval, by anyone whose cough is productive, or who is simultaneously using other nervous system depressants, such as sedatives, sleeping pills or antihistamines. However small its dosage, the codeine will boost another depressant's effect. Codeine-based cough suppressants are also dangerous for anyone suffering from a chronic pulmonary disorder such as asthma or emphysema—codeine dries out mucus tissue, and that effect will aggravate such ailments.

A safe substitute for codeine in most people is dextromethorphan, a synthetic drug with actions on the cough center that are similar to those of codeine though somewhat less powerful. Balancing this one slight disadvantage are sizable bonuses: Dextromethorphan is not addictive, and it provides a prolonged antitussive effect that may last up to eight hours—an especially valuable benefit if coughing interferes

## The cost of fighting colds

Although the best a cold remedy can do is ease symptoms without curing the illness, that relief is worth a lot to victims. Americans spent more than $1.5 billion in 1979 for nonprescription pills, potions and sprays that ameliorate discomforts, according to figures compiled by Arthur Weil of *Product Marketing* magazine. Expenditures in other industrialized countries were not far behind.

As indicated by the chart at right, which lists a year's sales of common nonprescription drugs in the United States, aspirin and aspirin substitutes make up almost two thirds of the total; these medicines, of course, are also used by people who do not have colds. So are allergy-relief medicines. But even if the sales for those items were cut in half, the total U.S. cold-fighting bill would still exceed one billion dollars—about five dollars for every American man, woman and child. Japan's total expenditure in 1979 was slightly more than four dollars a person, Australia's about three dollars.

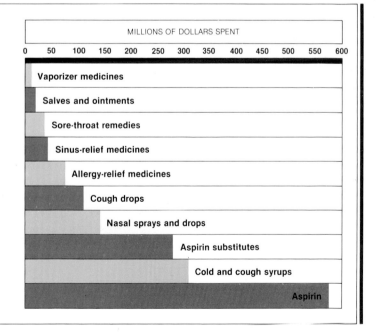

with sleep. But like all drugs, it brings its own side effects. Among them are occasional drowsiness, dizziness, mental confusion and digestive disorders; in very high dosages—well above the recommended amounts—it can also depress respiration, a dangerous effect for anyone suffering from such chronic lung disorders as emphysema.

The Cold and Cough Remedies Panel found that cough suppressants containing hydrocodone bitartrate and oil of turpentine were unsafe, ineffective or mislabeled, and it called for further study of 13 other ingredients. One of them, a derivative of opium called noscapine, is used in a few commercial products; in tests conducted by the American Pharmaceutical Association, noscapine won an endorsement as ''apparently safe at currently available OTC dosages, but effectiveness has not yet been proven.''

Expectorants, used to enhance the effects of productive coughs, are supposed to liquefy the sticky secretions normally produced by the mucous membrane lining the respiratory tract; in theory, they also decrease the viscosity of mucus obstructing the throat and larynx, so that it can be coughed up and expelled from the body. The most common substances employed for this purpose are chemicals such as ammonium chloride, SSKI (saturated solution of potassium iodide), guaifenesin and guaiacolate; all have occasional side effects ranging from stomach upset and vomiting to occasional disorders of the liver, kidneys and heart. Another expectorant chemical, terpin hydrate, which acts directly on the mucous membrane, is generally compounded in an elixir with high alcohol content. In the opinion of the review panel, none of these expectorants has any proved value in loosening mucus or relieving coughs. Moreover, the panel found a number of other expectorant agents not only ineffective but unsafe; among them are several materials derived from plants and long used for coughs, including an Oriental variety of the herb squill and the South American creeper ipecac.

The sensible course in treating a cough is fairly simple. Let a productive cough pretty much alone; an occasional hot beverage will help to loosen things up. For a dry cough, suck on some ordinary hard candy; medicated cough drops are little more than an expensive variant of hard candy, with no additional therapeutic value—the ''medication'' generally consists of an antiseptic, a cough suppressant or a mild local anesthetic. If the candy does not stimulate enough moisture to calm the cough, try a cough suppressant. Most are made up in a sweet syrup, and diabetics should check with their physicians before taking these cough remedies. They may contain sugar and alcohol, generally proscribed from diabetics' diets, and many also include decongestants, which act to increase sugar in the blood.

### Relief for aches and sore muscles

A final set of symptoms that may be associated with colds—fever, plus pain in one part of the body or another—is even more easily treated. The drug that most people most often take for a cold is the old reliable analgesic, aspirin, or its newer substitute, acetaminophen (best known by one of its trade names, Tylenol). Both come in numerous forms and under dozens of names, but all aspirins and acetaminophens are essentially the same, grain for grain. When you choose a painkiller, your choice should turn upon the issue of how well your body responds to one type or the other. Once this has been established, use the product that gives you the most grains or milligrams for your money.

Aspirin, the ingredient that, as the slogan of one brand proclaims, doctors recommend most, has been called the world's first wonder drug. Though the modern synthesized, mass-produced drug was not introduced until 1899, crude extracts containing compounds similar to the active ingredient in aspirin—a type of compound called a salicylate—have been prescribed for at least 2,000 years. Hippocrates, the father of Greek medicine, recommended the chewing of willow bark, which contains salicylates, to counter pain and reduce fever, and in many parts of the world willow- and poplar-bark teas have been brewed as painkillers for ages.

In 1971, researchers at The Royal College of Surgeons' Institute of Basic Medical Sciences in London discovered that the salicylates relieve pain by inhibiting the formation of substances called prostaglandins, produced by the body in response to a wide range of disorders, including inflammation. The discovery provided the key to aspirin's versatility.

# Do-it-yourself treatment at a college clinic

At the University of Wisconsin at Stevens Point, one course lasts only a few minutes, but its lesson is good for a lifetime. Each day about 50 sneezing, coughing students who show up at the campus health center are referred to the Cold Clinic — a group of plywood booths where the students, following printed instructions, learn to examine themselves, evaluate their symptoms and even choose most of their own medicines. The student with a typical mild cold can manage his illness without even talking to a physician or a nurse.

In one booth *(below, right-hand booth)* the student takes his own temperature with an electronic thermometer. He places a disposable cover over a probe, inserts the probe under his tongue, then reads the number of degrees flashing on a wall display panel.

Next, he examines his throat *(overleaf)* for inflammation or for the white spots that hint of bacterial infection. In another booth is posted a list of symptoms indicating an illness that is more serious than a cold; anyone suffering such symptoms is directed to drop out of line and consult a professional member of the university health center staff.

The do-it-yourself approach to cold care is a boon for overburdened health care personnel, who would otherwise face an "endless routine of explaining colds and sore throats," said Dr. John Betinis, designer and builder of the Stevens Point clinic. At the University of Massachusetts, where a similar program was established in 1975, requests for professional appointments from students with colds have been reduced by half.

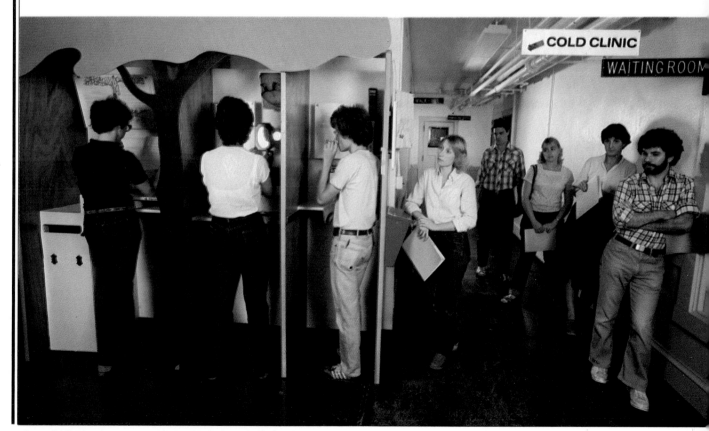

*Three students examine themselves and determine their own treatment in the booths of the Cold Clinic at the University of Wisconsin at Stevens Point, while others wait their turns. A series of wall signs tells them how to examine themselves and judge the severity of their own cold symptoms.*

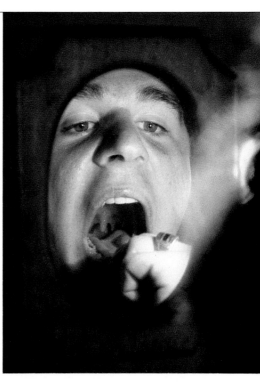

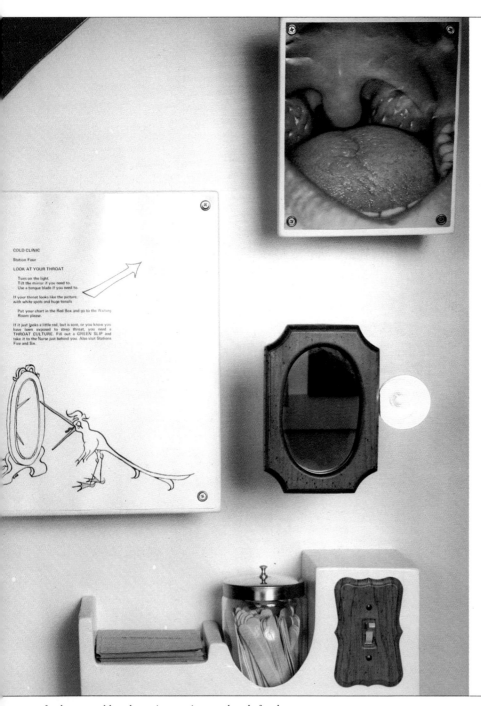

COLD CLINIC

Station Four

LOOK AT YOUR THROAT

Turn on the light.
Tilt the mirror if you need to.
Use a tongue blade if you need to.

If your throat looks like the picture,
with white spots and huge tonsils

Put your chart in the Red Box and go to the Waiting
Room please.

If it just looks a little red, but is sore, or you know you
have been exposed to strep throat, you need a
THROAT CULTURE. Fill out a GREEN SLIP and
take it to the Nurse just behind you. Also visit Stations
Five and Six.

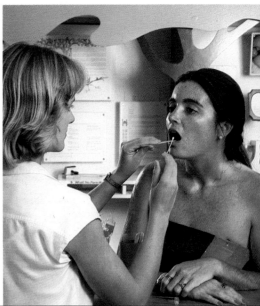

*In the second booth are instructions and tools for throat examination. Adjusting the angle of the high-intensity lamp and using a tongue depressor from the jar on the shelf, a student looks in the mirror. If his throat is as inflamed as the one pictured on the wall, he consults a staff member; for lesser symptoms, he may fill out a green slip (bottom) to request a throat culture.*

*Concerned by the appearance of her throat in the mirror (top), a student has her throat swabbed by a nurse, who remains on call when the clinic is open. Analysis of the student's throat culture will determine if she has a strep infection.*

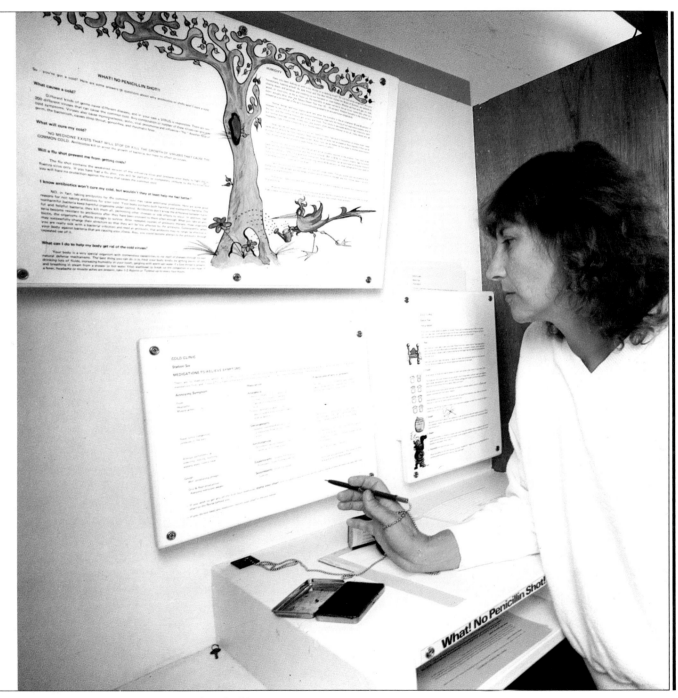

*At the last stop, a student scrutinizes a list of cold symptoms
and advice for easing them. The rubber stamp at her right hand
prints a form on which she can order nonprescription drugs
from the health center pharmacy. Other signs tell why penicillin is
useless against cold viruses, and counsel resting, drinking
fluids, gargling with warm salt water and humidifying room air.*

Inflammation of the mucous membrane is, of course, an early and prolonged symptom of a cold, and inflammation frequently causes fever, aching and soreness; aspirin is, therefore, the most appropriate and effective treatment for almost all the severe discomforts of colds.

Unfortunately, aspirin has side effects that make it unsuitable in some circumstances. It is acidic and has a tendency to irritate the lining of the stomach, making it unsuitable for anyone who has stomach ulcers or chronic gastric irritation, or who is taking prescription drugs for arthritis, some of which also cause stomach irritation. Aspirin has another acid effect important to gout sufferers; it slows down the excretion of uric acid, increasing the likelihood that uric acid will crystallize in the blood and bring on an attack of this painful ailment.

Aspirin is also an anticoagulant, slowing the clotting of blood. It will intensify the effect of other anticoagulants, often prescribed for heart patients. And it should be used with caution, if at all, by those for whom an increased tendency to bleed might be dangerous: hemophiliacs, pregnant women, women experiencing heavy menstrual flow, and anyone who expects to be operated on within a week.

Occasionally aspirin causes ringing in the ears, and it can send a tiny percentage of people into an allergic form of shock. In some analgesics, aspirin is combined with phenacetin, a stimulant; the phenacetin (not the aspirin) can cause kidney damage.

These side effects bother only a small minority of people—aspirin is a generally safe drug. However, if it is unsuitable, acetaminophen is the logical alternative. It rarely irritates the stomach or stimulates bleeding. Unlike aspirin, it does not reduce inflammation, so that its usefulness is somewhat limited for cold sufferers, and it does have a potentially dangerous side effect: Heavy doses can cause liver damage.

Aspirin and acetaminophen come in standard tablets of five grains, or about 300 milligrams, each; the usual recommended adult dosage is two tablets every three to four hours. ''Extra-strength'' products are simply tablets containing more than the standard measure of salicylates, but they are in no other way more powerful; you will get the same effect by taking more of the standard tablets. Buffered aspirin contains salts of magnesium or aluminum, which lessen the stomach upset caused by aspirin alone.

Some analgesics contain aspirin along with caffeine, alcohol and ascorbic acid. None of these combinations has proved its superiority over plain aspirin in the treatment of colds, and the superfluous ingredients may produce unwanted side effects. In addition, some multiaction cold medications contain substantial amounts of aspirin. If you are taking one of these catchall compounds, do not also take straight aspirin; you will exceed the recommended dose.

Another objection to the extensive use of aspirin for colds, though still theoretical, is surprising. The cold discomforts countered by aspirin—fever and muscle aches—are caused by the body's defensive reaction to the infection, and thus the effects of aspirin in easing those discomforts may well come about through inhibition of the defense. Some scientists believe that aspirin may retard the production of interferon and the inflammation responses, for example.

**Soothing a sore throat**

Ordinary analgesics such as aspirin have no effect on the sore throat that sometimes accompanies a cold—it may indeed be an inflammation of the mucous membrane in the throat caused by viral infection. A host of manufacturers claim to treat it successfully with over-the-counter remedies such as lozenges, mouthwashes and gargles. Some of them ease soreness, dryness or pain. But none of them cure the cause of the irritation. Many are ineffective and some add an irritant effect of their own.

One of the most common medications intended for sore throat is benzocaine, an anesthetic similar to the novocaine used by dentists. Like novocaine, it temporarily deadens the nerve endings that produce the sensations of pain. But according to the American Pharmaceutical Association, benzocaine must be present in concentrations of 5 to 20 per cent to give any prolonged benefit, and no over-the-counter product contains this concentration; several, however, contain enough to cause stomach upset or vomiting in some people.

Phenol and sodium phenolate, two other common sore-

## Why flying sometimes hurts the ears

Every air traveler knows the sensation of "popping" in the ears that occurs when an aircraft descends quickly. The popping does not last long—unless the passenger has a cold. Then it may bring hours of pain or virtual deafness. More lasting damage is rare but possible.

The problem is in the Eustachian tube, one and a half inches long, between the nose and the middle ear *(below)*. The tube is a vent, equalizing air pressure inside the middle ear with that outside. A cold swells nasal membranes and chokes off the tube, and when air pressure outside the ear changes abruptly, the choked tube cannot balance the pressure. The eardrum is moved sharply and stretched so that it hurts and cannot properly respond to sound vibrations.

The simplest way to open a blocked tube is to swallow and yawn, but these methods may not work for an airborne cold victim. Nasal spray or decongestant cold tablets, taken an hour or so before the plane begins its descent, may shrink the nasal membranes enough to unstop the Eustachian tube.

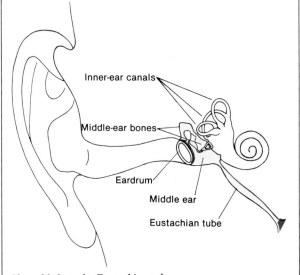

Inner-ear canals

Middle-ear bones

Eardrum

Middle ear

Eustachian tube

*If a cold shuts the Eustachian tube,*
*the blockage (blue) prevents balancing of air*
*pressure. In a descending airplane,*
*high pressure outside the ear causes painful*
*distortion of the eardrum (red). The*
*hearing bones and canals remain unaffected.*

throat remedies, deaden nerves, though very briefly, and may kill bacteria as well. But bacteria killers are useless in fighting viruses, and because phenol and sodium phenolate are often present in medicinal mouthwashes that contain alcohol or some other drying agent, their over-the-counter forms may actually contribute to the dryness that makes a sore throat feel so wretched. The American Pharmaceutical Association, which has an interest in promoting over-the-counter sore-throat treatments, recently added another count to the indictment against these substances. In a handbook for the profession, the association reminded its members that any change in the bacteria normally present in the body could have adverse effects: "It is possible that alteration of the normal oral cavity flora actually may allow invasion by pathogenic organisms," leading to other infections.

What, then, should you do for a sore throat? First, be sure that the cause of the soreness is indeed a cold. A wide variety of irritants and ailments other than viruses can be at fault, from heavy cigarette smoking, spicy foods and air pollution to infection by streptococcal bacteria—strep throat—tonsillitis and even throat cancer. One test is duration. A sore throat caused by a constant irritant such as smoking or air pollution will cure itself in a few days if the irritant is removed; a condition, even a mild one, that lasts more than two weeks is almost certainly due to more than a cold. Another test is severity and associated symptoms. The pain of strep throat, for example, can be severe, and is accompanied by swollen glands and white or yellowish pus spots at the back of the throat. If at any time while you have a sore throat your temperature rises sharply, or if you develop a rash (a symptom of both infectious mononucleosis and scarlet fever), or see spots at the back of your throat or have any other symptoms not readily attributable to a cold, consult your doctor.

If what you have is a sore throat associated with the runny nose, stuffiness, coughing and sneezing of a true cold, then lozenges, troches and gargles may offer some relief. The medicated candies have something of an edge. Gargles—whether medicated or simply the old home remedy of warm salt water—reach only a small portion of the throat, near its entrance; when you gargle, your throat automatically con-

# When a cold is not a cold

| DISEASE | COLD SYMPTOMS | | | | | | | | | | ADDITIONAL SYMPTOMS |
|---|---|---|---|---|---|---|---|---|---|---|---|
| | Stuffy or runny nose | Sneezing | Fever | Sore throat | Cough | Headache | Nonspecific discomfort | Muscle pain | Chills | Nausea | |
| ALLERGY | ● | ● | | ● | ● | | | | | | Itchy eyes; noisy or difficult breathing |
| BRONCHITIS | | | ● | | ● | | ● | ● | | | Chest pain when coughing; difficult breathing; wheezing; increasing breathlessness |
| DIPHTHERIA (mainly in children) | | | ● | ● | | | | | | | High fever (102° F. or above); exhaustion; bad breath; difficult breathing or swallowing |
| GERMAN MEASLES | ● | | ● | | | ● | | | | ● | Inflamed eyes; body rash after about the fourth day |
| LEGIONNAIRE'S DISEASE (mainly in men over 40) | | | ● | | ● | ● | ● | ● | | | Cough with rust-colored mucus; diarrhea; pain around the rib cage |
| MEASLES | ● | | ● | ● | ● | | | | | | Inflamed eyes; white spots inside the cheeks; rash, spreading from face to trunk and limbs |
| MENINGITIS | | | ● | | | ● | | ● | | | Increasingly severe headache; sensitivity to light; convulsions |
| MONONUCLEOSIS | ● | | ● | ● | ● | ● | ● | | | | Extremely sore throat; swelling from chin to ear; pain just above the genital area |
| MUMPS | | | ● | ● | | ● | ● | | | | Swollen neck glands; pain behind the ears; difficult swallowing |
| PNEUMONIA | | | ● | | ● | ● | | ● | | | Painful cough; cough that produces rust-colored mucus; difficult breathing |
| POLIOMYELITIS | | | ● | | | ● | | ● | | | Muscle cramps or spasms; extremely stiff neck; weakness in the arms and legs; sensitivity to light; diarrhea |
| SCARLET FEVER | | | ● | ● | | ● | ● | | | ● | Red rash on trunk and limbs; abdominal pain |
| STREP THROAT | | | ● | ● | | ● | | | ● | | Difficult swallowing; thick white or yellow mucus at the back of the throat |
| WHOOPING COUGH (mainly in children) | ● | ● | | ● | ● | | ● | | | | Noisy or difficult breathing; violent paroxysms of coughing, with as many as eight to ten coughs in one breath, ending in a loud crow or whoop; bluish complexion |

Many diseases, some of them serious, first appear in the guise of a cold. It can be especially difficult to distinguish influenza from a cold, because the two share so many symptoms (page 99). But several other ailments can begin with signs no more ominous than those of a cold—a cough or stuffed-up nose. When such symptoms are joined by others less familiar—a rash, for example, or a swelling—something more than a cold is probably assailing your body, and you should consult a physician. The chart above describes 14 illnesses that may, especially in the early stage, be mistaken for a cold. The cold-mimicking symptoms are indicated by black dots; the additional signs that point to the true illness are described in detail.

stricts, preventing the liquid medication from coming into contact with the lower throat tissue.

Lozenges and troches are the same—cough drops with a little anesthetic added—except for their shapes, which give them their names. Lozenges are angular—the word "lozenge" is an old term for a "diamond shape." Troches are disks and derive their name from a Greek word meaning "wheel." When either type is left to dissolve at the back of the mouth, a certain amount of the soothing material will drip down into the throat. The trouble is that, even in this form, the amount has little therapeutic value.

More effective than any attempt to cure a sore throat are steps to prevent further irritation of the membranes. If you are a smoker, stop smoking. To rest your throat, talk as little as possible. Eat bland foods and drink comfortably hot liquids such as broth and tea. Raise the room's humidity to 50 per cent or more with a vaporizer.

**A medicine chest for colds**

By now you may have resolved to go through your medicine cabinet for a skeptical look at what you have on hand for coughs and colds. You probably have much more than you need. Begin by reading labels, looking for products containing chemicals that are irrelevant to the relief of colds, and for warnings that might apply to you or members of your family. Check bottles and packages for expiration dates and get rid of outdated drugs. Be sure that the drug containers are airtight; those small, flat aspirin tins, for example, fail this test.

When you are finished, you should be down to a few basics: a bottle of standard aspirin, if everyone in the household can tolerate aspirin; if not, acetaminophen. Add decongestant, unopened, and a cough suppressant. If there are children in your family, you should have medicines formulated for them. Small bottles and packages are generally better than large. Though they are a little more costly dose for dose, you are better off renewing the products regularly as you use them up; and nasal sprays and drops, which soon become contaminated through use, should always be bought in personal-sized dispensers and discarded when a cold has run its course. While you are going through the medicine

cabinet, make sure that you have an oral thermometer and, for young children, a rectal thermometer as well.

A final word of caution: Colds and the coughs associated with colds are self-limiting diseases. Their normal duration is seven to 10 days, with gradual improvement typically appearing around the fourth or fifth day. Because they are relatively mild ailments of limited duration, many physicians think they should not be treated with any drugs at all. The medicines available do not fight the diseases so much as ease their symptoms; thus they make you feel better than you really are and encourage you to continue your normal routine—and spread viruses further. In this way, cold remedies may cause more people to get sick than otherwise would.

By curbing symptoms, cold medicines may also deceive you, making you believe a more serious illness is only a cold. No matter what medication you use, do not take over-the-counter remedies beyond the sixth or seventh day after the onset of symptoms. Watch for symptoms of greater danger.

Cold symptoms that last too long or that include severe pain in the sinuses or the ears require professional attention. The same applies to cold symptoms accompanied by fever that continues longer than three days or becomes very high—more than 102° in an adult, 103° in a child. Similarly, a deep, racking cough, chest pains and labored breathing are evidences of a problem that is beyond self-medication. Other atypical and threatening symptoms include: a rash, swollen neck glands, pus at the back of the throat, nausea, severe headaches, and stiffness and pain in the back of the neck that make it almost impossible to touch chin to chest. These symptoms could indicate measles, mumps, strep throat, polio or meningitis—any of which may first appear as nose or throat discomfort.

Obviously, cold symptoms can be deceptive; whenever you feel them, follow the course of your ailment carefully. If what seems like a cold lasts longer than two weeks, if you find yourself becoming increasingly worse instead of better, or if you develop such complications as earaches, shortness of breath, prolonged high fever, swollen glands in your neck, bloody sputum, a painful sore throat or a painful and persistent cough, consult a physician promptly. ✳

# How to choose the medicines that work

No drug can cure a cold, but some drugs do relieve its symptoms. For the most part, these drugs can be bought without a doctor's prescription, and their manufacturers tell the world about them in an avalanche of advertising. But in attempting to treat a cold, you should be aware of certain pitfalls and perils of self-medication.

The table on the following pages lists the most commonly used cold drugs by their generic chemical names; brand names are listed on pages 94-95. When shopping for a drug, read the labels to find the generic names in the first column of the table. The second column lists the intended or claimed effects of each drug: Choose the medicine that produces the effect you need. Many brands are "shotgun remedies," which combine two or more drugs in an attempt to relieve all the common symptoms of a cold. But colds differ from one sufferer to another, and so do their symptoms; generally, you will be better off buying remedies containing only the ingredients that treat your particular set of symptoms.

Even then, you cannot always be sure that the effect claimed for a drug is actually produced in the user. The drugs listed in the table have all been studied by a U.S. Food and Drug Administration advisory review panel, which found all the drugs reasonably safe ("if," in the familiar phrase, "used as directed") but not equally effective. In some cases, they may not be effective at all.

All drugs have side effects, and every side effect is a potential danger. Use the third and fourth columns of the table to check the minor and major side effects of any medicine you plan to take. And use the column on special cautions to find possible dangers that are not side effects of a medicine when it is used alone, but may arise when the medicine is taken along with other medicines, alcohol, tobacco, sedatives and the like.

Whatever course of medication you decide upon, monitor your symptoms closely. If the drugs you take do not relieve the symptoms of a cold in two or three days, see a doctor.

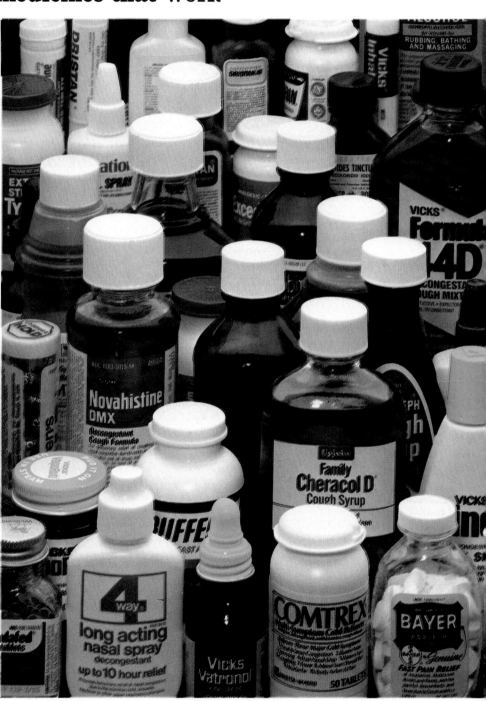

*The patent medicines above are a small sampling of the hundreds sold for coughs and colds. None cure, but most contain active ingredients that will relieve cold symptoms. To choose the products that treat your symptoms most effectively, find the ingredients on the labels or in the index on pages 94-95, then check their effects in the table beginning at right.*

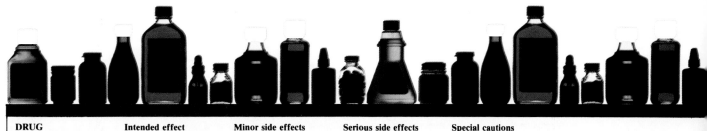

| DRUG | Intended effect | Minor side effects | Serious side effects | Special cautions |
|---|---|---|---|---|
| **ACETAMINOPHEN** | Relieves headaches and neuralgia; relieves mild to moderate pain in muscles and joints; lowers fever | Dizziness; diarrhea and upset stomach after slight overdose | Liver damage or hepatitis; reduced white-blood-cell and platelet count; disturbed bone-marrow functions | Do not take if you have kidney or liver disease. Overdose can cause liver damage, especially in young children. Consult doctor if you develop sore throat, unusual bleeding or unusual bruising, three signs of bone-marrow disorder. Consult doctor if symptoms are not relieved in 3 days or if they recur repeatedly. |
| **AMMONIUM CHLORIDE** | Loosens and increases respiratory-tract secretions, making them easier to cough up | Upset stomach; vomiting | Large doses occasionally toxic to victims of kidney, liver or heart disease | The FDA has been unable to determine the effectiveness of this drug. Consult doctor before taking if you have lung, kidney, liver or heart disease. Consult doctor if you have persistent cough. |
| **ASPIRIN** | Relieves headaches and neuralgia; relieves mild to moderate pain in muscles and joints; lowers fever; reduces inflammation | Upset stomach; ringing in the ears; mild drowsiness | Bleeding and erosion of the stomach lining; gastric ulcer may develop or be activated with prolonged use; liver and kidney damage; slowed blood clotting | Take with caution if you have hay fever or asthma—you may have an allergic reaction marked by nasal congestion, wheezing or shock. Stop taking 1 week before surgery unless otherwise directed. Consult doctor before taking if you have bleeding disorders, are taking drugs to prevent blood clots, have an ulcer or are pregnant. Aspirin may alter the effects of drugs given for arthritis, gout and diabetes. Notify doctor if you feel any effects of drug interaction. Do not take tablets that smell like vinegar—the odor indicates the presence of acetic acid, a by-product of aspirin decomposition that can irritate the mouth and stomach. Minimize stomach irritation by taking with a glass of milk or water. |
| **BELLADONNA ALKALOIDS** | Dries and shrinks nasal and throat membranes | Blurred vision; drowsiness; dry mouth and throat; reduced perspiration | Chronic and severe constipation; behavioral disturbances, including confusion, agitation and inappropriate actions; acute glaucoma; difficult breathing; difficult urinating; hepatitis; skin rash; reduced blood-platelet count | The FDA has been unable to determine the effectiveness of this drug. Consult doctor before taking if you have glaucoma, intestinal disease or an enlarged prostate. Consult your doctor if you develop unusual bruising or bleeding, two signs of reduced blood-platelet count. Do not take with alcohol or other depressants. Drowsiness can make driving or operating heavy machinery dangerous. Reduced perspiration can make exercising or working in hot weather dangerous. |

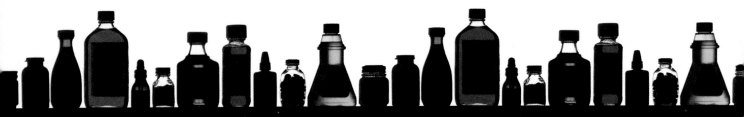

| DRUG | Intended effect | Minor side effects | Serious side effects | Special cautions |
|---|---|---|---|---|
| **BENZOCAINE** | Relieves sore throat pain | Upset stomach; vomiting; skin rash | None | Consult doctor for a severe sore throat, especially in a child under 6. A sore throat can spread infection into the middle ear and brain; a strep throat can lead to rheumatic fever or kidney disease. |
| **BROMPHENIRAMINE** | Dries and shrinks nasal membranes | Dry mouth and throat; drowsiness; dizziness; thickening of the bronchial secretions; upset stomach; loss of appetite | Disturbed bone-marrow functions; reduced white-blood-cell count; rise in blood sugar; difficult urinating | Do not take with alcohol or other depressants. Consult doctor before taking if you have glaucoma or difficulty urinating or plan to have surgery in the near future. Consult your doctor if you develop sore throat, unusual bleeding or unusual bruising, three signs of bone-marrow disorder. Consult doctor if drug causes nervousness and tremors, particularly in young children. Drowsiness can make driving or operating heavy machinery dangerous. |
| **CAMPHOR** | Dries and shrinks nasal membranes; loosens and increases respiratory-tract secretions, making them easier to cough up | Skin irritation or numbness; nausea; vomiting | None | The FDA has been unable to determine the effectiveness of this drug. Do not rub ointment vigorously into the skin; it can cause local irritation. Keep ointment out of reach of young children; it can cause convulsions if taken by mouth. |
| **CHLORPHENIRAMINE** | Action similar to BROMPHENIRAMINE | | | |
| **CODEINE or CODEINE SULFATE or CODEINE PHOSPHATE** | Suppresses coughing; relieves mild to moderate pain | Constipation; loss of appetite; upset stomach; drowsiness; skin rash; dizziness | Slowed heartbeat; nervousness, especially in children; physical and psychological dependence with prolonged use; difficult breathing | Consult doctor if you suffer from liver, lung, kidney or thyroid disease or plan to have surgery. Do not take with alcohol or other depressants. Consult doctor if you are pregnant; codeine may affect the functions of an embryo or, during labor, impair the breathing of an infant. Drowsiness can make driving or operating heavy machinery dangerous. Consult doctor before taking if you have a history of drug abuse; codeine is a narcotic. |
| **DEXTROMETHOR-PHAN** | Suppresses coughing | Drowsiness; dizziness; upset stomach; vomiting | None | Consult doctor if your cough brings up fluid. Drowsiness can make driving or operating heavy machinery dangerous. Some cough syrups have a high alcohol content, which can cause oversedation. |

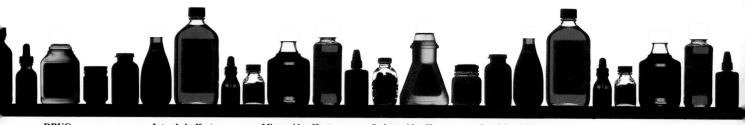

| DRUG | Intended effect | Minor side effects | Serious side effects | Special cautions |
|------|----------------|-------------------|---------------------|-----------------|
| **DOXYLAMINE** | Dries and shrinks nasal membranes | Drowsiness; dizziness; dry mouth and throat; thickening of bronchial secretions; upset stomach; loss of appetite; headache; skin rash; sweating; rapid heartbeat | Difficult urinating; behavioral disturbances, including confusion, agitation and inappropriate actions | Consult doctor if you have glaucoma, asthma or peptic ulcers, if you plan to have surgery in the near future or if you have difficulty in urinating. Drowsiness can make driving or operating heavy machinery dangerous. Some cough syrups have a high alcohol content, which can cause oversedation. |
| **EPHEDRINE** | Dries and shrinks nasal membranes | Nervousness; insomnia; headache; upset stomach; constipation; loss of appetite; rapid heartbeat; dizziness; feeling of warmth; reduced perspiration | Difficult urinating; rise in blood pressure and blood sugar; behavioral disturbances, including confusion, agitation and inappropriate actions | Do not take with alcohol or other depressants. Consult doctor before taking if you have heart or thyroid disease, glaucoma, high blood pressure or diabetes, plan to have surgery in the near future or have difficulty in urinating. Do not take with monoamine oxidase (MAO) inhibitors; the combination can cause a dangerous rise in blood pressure. Do not take with digitalis; the combination can disturb the heart rhythm. Do not give to children under 6, or to people 60 or over; the drug can disturb the heart rhythm. Reduced perspiration can make exercising or working in hot weather dangerous. |
| **EUCALYPTOL or EUCALYPTUS OIL** | Suppresses coughing; loosens and increases respiratory-tract secretions, making them easier to cough up | Nausea; vomiting | Dizziness, weakness and stupor after large doses | The FDA has been unable to determine the effectiveness of this drug. Do not use ointment on broken skin or in or on the nostrils; it can cause skin irritation and may be absorbed rapidly into the blood, where it is toxic. Consult doctor before applying ointment to children under 6; it is easily absorbed into the blood. |
| **GUAIFENESIN** | Loosens and increases respiratory-tract secretions, making them easier to cough up | Upset stomach; vomiting; occasional drowsiness | None | The FDA has been unable to determine the effectiveness of this drug. Consult doctor if you have persistent cough. |
| **IPECAC SYRUP** | Loosens and increases respiratory-tract secretions, making them easier to cough up | Upset stomach; vomiting | None | The FDA has been unable to determine the effectiveness of this drug. Consult doctor if you have persistent cough. Do not take longer than 1 week. Do not give to children under 6; a child may be choked by loosened secretions. |

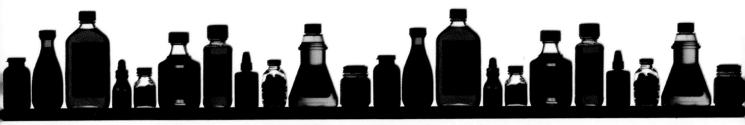

| DRUG | Intended effect | Minor side effects | Serious side effects | Special cautions |
|---|---|---|---|---|
| **LEVODESOXYEPHE-DRINE** | Dries and shrinks nasal membranes | Burning, dryness and stinging of the nasal membranes; rebound effect after extended use, with renewed congestion that may be worse than the original condition; nervousness; insomnia; headache; blurred vision | Rise in blood pressure and blood sugar | To avoid rebound effect, do not take longer than 4 days. Consult doctor before taking if you have heart or thyroid disease, high blood pressure or diabetes or plan to have surgery in the near future. |
| **MENTHOL** | Loosens and increases respiratory-tract secretions, making them easier to cough up; suppresses coughing; temporary relief of sore-throat pain | Nausea, vomiting and dizziness after large dose; skin and eye irritation | Coma after large oral doses; difficult breathing in infants after inhalation; death after oral doses of 2 grams or more of menthol | The FDA has been unable to determine the effectiveness of this drug. Do not apply directly to the nostrils of children under 2; it can cause throat spasms. Consult doctor for severe sore throat, especially in a .child under 6. A sore throat can spread infection into the middle ear and brain; a strep throat can lead to rheumatic fever or kidney disease. Do not use ointment on broken skin or in or on the nostrils; in such areas it can cause local skin irritation and may be absorbed rapidly into the blood, where it is toxic. Consult doctor before applying ointment to children under 6; it is easily absorbed into the blood. |
| **NAPHAZOLINE** | Dries and shrinks nasal membranes | Burning, dryness and stinging of the nasal membranes; rebound effect after extended use, with renewed congestion that may be worse than the original condition; nervousness; insomnia; headache; blurred vision | Rise in blood pressure and blood sugar; disturbances of heart rhythm | Consult doctor before taking if you have heart disease, high blood pressure, glaucoma, diabetes or hyperthyroidism. Do not use in atomizers with aluminum parts because it interacts with this metal, causing the drug to break down. Do not take with monoamine oxidase (MAO) inhibitors; the combination can cause a dangerous rise in blood pressure. Consult doctor before giving to children under 6; an overdose can cause coma and slow the heart rate. To avoid rebound effect, do not take for more than 4 days. |
| **NOSCAPINE** | Suppresses coughing | Drowsiness; headache; dizziness; upset stomach; skin rash | None | The FDA has been unable to determine the effectiveness of this drug. |

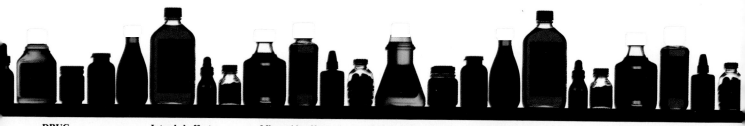

| DRUG | Intended effect | Minor side effects | Serious side effects | Special cautions |
|---|---|---|---|---|
| OXYMETAZOLINE | Dries and shrinks nasal membranes | Burning, dryness and stinging of the nasal membranes; rebound effect after extended use, with renewed congestion; nervousness; insomnia; headache; blurred vision | Rise in blood pressure, heart rate and blood sugar after large doses | Consult your doctor before taking if you have heart disease, high blood pressure, diabetes or hyperthyroidism. Do not take with monoamine oxidase (MAO) inhibitors; the combination can cause a dangerous rise in blood pressure. To avoid rebound effect, do not take for more than 4 days. |
| PHENIRAMINE | Dries and shrinks nasal membranes | Drowsiness; weakness; dry mouth and throat; constipation; skin rash; headaches; nervousness; blurred vision; vomiting; upset stomach; diarrhea | Emotional and behavioral disturbances, including confusion, agitation and inappropriate actions; difficult urinating | Consult doctor before taking if you are 60 or older; emotional and behavioral disturbances occur most frequently in the elderly. Drowsiness can make driving or operating heavy machinery dangerous. Do not take with alcohol or other depressants. Consult doctor before taking if you have glaucoma or plan to have surgery in the near future. Consult doctor if you develop difficulty urinating or if drug causes nervousness and tremors, particularly in young children. |
| PHENOL | Relieves sore-throat pain | Upset stomach and vomiting with large dose | Decreased blood pressure and difficult urinating with overdose | Consult doctor if severe sore throat occurs, especially in a child under 6. A sore throat can spread infection into the middle ear and brain; a strep throat can lead to rheumatic fever or kidney disease. |
| PHENYLEPHRINE | Dries and shrinks nasal membranes | Burning, dryness and stinging of the nasal membranes; rebound effect after extended use, with renewed congestion; nervousness; insomnia; headache | Changes in blood pressure and heartbeat with large doses | Consult doctor before taking if you have heart disease, high blood pressure, diabetes or hyperthyroidism. Do not take with monoamine oxidase (MAO) inhibitors or tricyclic antidepressants; the combination can cause a dangerous rise in blood pressure. To avoid rebound effect, do not take for more than 4 days. |
| PHENYLPROPANOL-AMINE | Dries and shrinks nasal membranes | Nervousness; insomnia; headache; upset stomach; dizziness; feeling of warmth | Changes in blood pressure and heartbeat; severe behavioral disturbances, including confusion, agitation and inappropriate actions; arrythmias and changes in heart rate | Consult doctor before taking if you have heart disease, glaucoma, high blood pressure, diabetes or difficulty urinating. Do not take with monoamine oxidase (MAO) inhibitors; the combination can cause a dangerous rise in blood pressure. Do not take with digitalis; the combination can disturb the heart rhythm. |

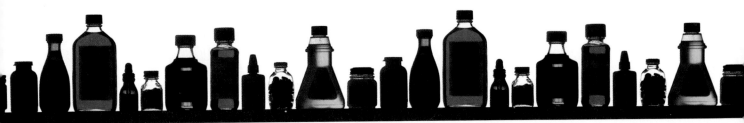

| DRUG | Intended effect | Minor side effects | Serious side effects | Special cautions |
|------|-----------------|--------------------|--------------------|------------------|
| **PHENYLTOLOX-AMINE** | Dries and shrinks nasal membranes | Upset stomach; diarrhea; heartburn; nausea; drowsiness | None | The FDA has been unable to determine the effectiveness of this drug.<br>Drowsiness can make driving or operating heavy machinery dangerous. |
| **PROPYLHEXEDRINE** | Dries and shrinks nasal membranes | Burning, dryness and stinging of the nasal membranes; rebound effect after extended use, with renewed congestion that may be worse than the original condition; nervousness; insomnia; headache; blurred vision; nausea | None | Consult doctor before taking if you have heart disease, glaucoma, diabetes or an overactive thyroid.<br>Do not take with monoamine oxidase (MAO) inhibitors or tricyclic antidepressants; the combination can cause a dangerous rise in blood pressure. |
| **PSEUDOEPHEDRINE** | Dries and shrinks nasal membranes | Nervousness; sweating; upset stomach; weakness; insomnia; vomiting; headache; reduced perspiration | Severe behavioral disturbances; rise in blood pressure; slowed heart rate; difficult urinating | Consult doctor before taking if you have heart or thyroid disease, glaucoma, high blood pressure or diabetes, if you plan to have surgery in the near future or if you have difficulty urinating.<br>Do not take with monoamine oxidase (MAO) inhibitors; the combination can cause a dangerous rise in blood pressure.<br>Do not take with digitalis; the combination can disturb the heart rhythm.<br>Reduced perspiration can make exercising or working in hot weather dangerous. |
| **PYRILAMINE** | Dries and shrinks nasal membranes | Sweating; dry mouth and throat; skin rash; blurred vision; headache; loss of appetite; nervousness; dizziness; drowsiness; insomnia; upset stomach; diarrhea | Difficult urinating; behavioral disturbances, including confusion, agitation and inappropriate actions | Do not take with alcohol or other depressants, which enhance the drug's depressive effect on the central nervous system.<br>Consult doctor before taking if you are 60 or over, plan to have surgery in the near future or have ulcers, asthma or difficulty urinating.<br>Drowsiness can make driving or operating heavy machinery dangerous. |
| **SODIUM CITRATE** | Loosens and increases respiratory-tract secretions, making them easier to cough up | Upset stomach; diarrhea | None | The FDA has been unable to determine the effectiveness of this drug.<br>Take with a glass of milk or water to minimize stomach irritation.<br>Consult doctor if you have heart or kidney disease or a persistent or chronic cough. |

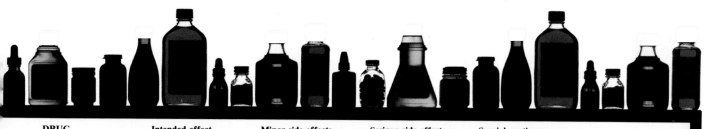

| DRUG | Intended effect | Minor side effects | Serious side effects | Special cautions |
|---|---|---|---|---|
| **SODIUM PHENOLATE** | Action similar to PHENOL | | | |
| **TERPIN HYDRATE** | Loosens and increases respiratory-tract secretions | Upset stomach; vomiting | None | The FDA has been unable to determine the effectiveness of this drug. Consult doctor before taking if you have a history of drug abuse; preparations with terpin hydrate usually contain high content of codeine, a narcotic drug. |
| **THENYLDIAMINE** | Dries and shrinks nasal membranes | Burning, dryness and stinging of the nasal membranes and throat; rebound effect after extended use, with renewed congestion | None | The FDA has been unable to determine the effectiveness of this drug. |
| **TURPENTINE OIL (Spirits of Turpentine)** | Loosens and increases respiratory-tract secretions, making them easier to cough up | Skin rash; itching; soreness | None | The FDA has been unable to determine the effectiveness of this drug. Do not take by mouth. The FDA has determined that turpentine oil is safe only when used as an ointment or in vaporizers; large oral doses have been followed by vomiting, diarrhea, acute generalized pain, bloody stools, kidney pain and degeneration of the liver. Do not use ointment on broken skin or in or on the nostrils; in such areas it can cause local skin irritation and may be absorbed rapidly into the blood, where it is toxic. Consult doctor before applying ointment to children under 6; it is easily absorbed into the blood. |
| **XYLOMETAZOLINE** | Dries and shrinks nasal membranes | Burning, dryness and stinging of the nasal membranes; rebound effect after extended use, with renewed congestion that may be worse than the original condition; nervousness; insomnia; headache; dizziness; blurred vision | Rises in blood pressure, heart rate and blood sugar | Consult doctor before taking if you have heart disease, high blood pressure, glaucoma, diabetes or hyperthyroidism. Do not take with monoamine oxidase (MAO) inhibitors; the combination can cause a dangerous rise in blood pressure. To avoid rebound effect, do not take for more than 4 days. |

## Index of brand names

Listed alphabetically on these pages are the brand names of 154 widely used nonprescription cold remedies. Following the name of each preparation are its active ingredients, identified by their generic chemical names; their properties are described in the table on pages 87-93. To use the list, first look up the name of a product and note its ingredients, then check those ingredients in the preceding table for their effects and side effects. Remember that remedies containing a number of active ingredients are not necessarily better than single-ingredient preparations; choose a product with ingredients that treat only the symptoms you suffer.

ACTOL EXPECTORANT: guaifenesin, noscapine

AFRIN NASAL SPRAY: oxymetazoline

ALCONEFRIN: phenylephrine

ALKA-SELTZER PLUS: aspirin, chlorpheniramine, phenylpropanolamine

ARRESTIN EXTRA STRENGTH COUGH MEDICINE: dextromethorphan, sodium citrate

ATUSSIN EXPECTORANT: chlorpheniramine, guaifenesin, phenylephrine, phenylpropanolamine

BAYER CHILDREN'S COLD TABLETS: aspirin, phenylpropanolamine

BAYER COUGH SYRUP FOR CHILDREN: dextromethorphan, phenylpropanolamine

BAYER DECONGESTANT COLD AND ALLERGY REMEDY: aspirin, chlorpheniramine, phenylpropanolamine

BENYLIN DM: dextromethorphan

BENZEDREX INHALER: menthol, propylhexedrine

BIOMYDRIN: phenylephrine

BREACOL: chlorpheniramine, dextromethorphan, phenylpropanolamine

BRONCHO-TUSSIN: codeine phosphate, terpin hydrate

BUFFERIN: aspirin

C3 CAPSULES: chlorpheniramine, dextromethorphan, phenylpropanolamine

CALCIDRINE SYRUP: codeine, ephedrine

CENAGESIC: phenylephrine, pyrilamine

CEPASTAT LOZENGES: eucalyptus oil, menthol, phenol

CHERACOL: codeine phosphate, guaifenesin

CHERACOL D COUGH SYRUP: dextromethorphan, guaifenesin

CHILDREN'S HOLD: dextromethorphan, phenylpropanolamine

CHLORASEPTIC DM COUGH CONTROL LOZENGES: dextromethorphan, phenol, sodium phenolate

CHLOR-TRIMETON EXPECTORANT: ammonium chloride, chlorpheniramine, guaifenesin, phenylephrine, sodium citrate

CHLOR-TRIMETON TABLETS: chlorpheniramine

CODIMAL CAPSULES OR TABLETS: acetaminophen, chlorpheniramine, pseudoephedrine

COLCHEK DECONGESTANT TABS: chlorpheniramine, dextromethorphan, phenylpropanolamine

COLREX CAPSULES: acetaminophen, chlorpheniramine,phenylephrine

COLREX SYRUP: chlorpheniramine, dextromethorphan, phenylephrine

COMTREX: acetaminophen, chlorpheniramine, dextromethorphan, phenylpropanolamine

CONGESPIRIN: aspirin, phenylephrine

CONSOTUSS: dextromethorphan, doxylamine

CONTAC: belladonna alkaloids, chlorpheniramine, phenylpropanolamine

CORICIDIN COUGH SYRUP: ammonium chloride, chlorpheniramine, guaifenesin, phenylpropanolamine

CORICIDIN D: aspirin, chlorpheniramine, phenylpropanolamine

CORICIDIN MEDILETS: chlorpheniramine

CORICIDIN TABLETS: aspirin, chlorpheniramine

CORYBAN-D COUGH SYRUP: acetaminophen, dextromethorphan, guaifenesin, phenylephrine

COSANYL COUGH SYRUP: codeine phosphate, pseudoephedrine

COTUSSIS: codeine phosphate, terpin hydrate

COTYLENOL COLD FORMULA TABLETS: acetaminophen, chlorpheniramine, phenylpropanolamine

COTYLENOL LIQUID COLD FORMULA: acetaminophen, chlorpheniramine, dextromethorphan, pseudoephedrine

COVANGESIC LIQUID AND TABLETS: acetaminophen, chlorpheniramine, phenylephrine, phenylpropanolamine, pyrilamine

CREOMULSION: ipecac, menthol

DATRIL: acetaminophen

DECAPRYN: doxylamine

DIMACOL LIQUID: dextromethorphan, guaifenesin, pseudoephedrine

DIMETANE: brompheniramine

DRISTAN-AF: acetaminophen, chlorpheniramine, phenylephrine

DRISTAN DECONGESTANT TABLETS: aspirin, chlorpheniramine, phenylephrine

DRISTAN INHALER: eucalyptol, menthol, propylhexedrine

DRISTAN LONG-LASTING NASAL MIST: xylometazoline

DRISTAN NASAL MIST: pheniramine, phenylephrine

DURAMIST PM NASAL SPRAY: xylometazoline

DURATION NASAL SPRAY: oxymetazoline

EXCEDRIN: acetaminophen

EXCEDRIN P.M.: acetaminophen, pyrilamine

EXTENDAC: belladonna alkaloids, chlorpheniramine, pheniramine, phenylpropanolamine

EXTRA STRENGTH TYLENOL: acetaminophen

4-WAY LONG-ACTING NASAL SPRAY: xylometazoline

4-WAY NASAL SPRAY: naphazoline, phenylephrine, pyrilamine

FIRST SIGN: pseudoephedrine

FORMULA 44 COUGH CONTROL DISCS: benzocaine, dextromethorphan, menthol

FORMULA 44 COUGH MIXTURE: dextromethorphan, doxylamine, sodium citrate

FORMULA 44-D: dextromethorphan, guaifenesin, phenylpropanolamine

HALLS: dextromethorphan, eucalyptus oil, menthol, phenylpropanolamine

HISTADYL EC: ammonium chloride, codeine phosphate, ephedrine, menthol

HOLD: dextromethorphan

HOLD COUGH SYRUP: dextromethorphan, phenylpropanolamine

IPSATOL: ammonium chloride, ipecac syrup

I-SEDRIN PLAIN: ephedrine

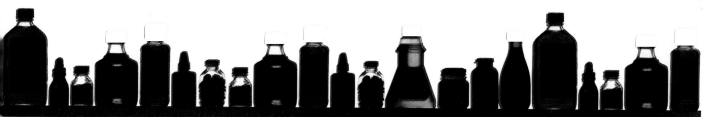

LISTERINE COUGH CONTROL LOZENGES: benzocaine, dextromethorphan
MENTHOLATUM OINTMENT: eucalyptus oil, menthol, turpentine oil
MENTHOL CHLORASEPTIC LIQUID OR SPRAY: menthol, phenol,
   sodium phenolate
MULTI-SYMPTOM: brompheniramine, dextromethorphan, pseudoephedrine
NTZ: phenylephrine, thenyldiamine
NALDETUSS: acetaminophen, dextromethorphan, phenylpropanolamine,
   phenyltoloxamine
NEOPHIBAN TABLETS: acetaminophen, guaifenesin, phenylpropanolamine,
   phenyltoloxamine
NEO-SYNEPHRINE COMPOUND: acetaminophen, phenylephrine,
   thenyldiamine
NEO-SYNEPHRINE II NASAL SPRAY: xylometazoline
NORATUSS: ammonium chloride, codeine phosphate, terpin hydrate
NOVAFED: pseudoephedrine
NOVAHISTINE DH: codeine phosphate, phenylpropanolamine
NOVAHISTINE DMX: dextromethorphan, guaifenesin, pseudoephedrine
NOVAHISTINE ELIXIR: chlorpheniramine, phenylpropanolamine
NOVAHISTINE EXPECTORANT: chlorpheniramine, codeine phosphate,
   guaifenesin, phenylpropanolamine
NYQUIL NIGHTTIME COLDS MEDICINE: acetaminophen,
   dextromethorphan, doxylamine, ephedrine
ORNACOL CAPSULES AND LIQUID: dextromethorphan,
   phenylpropanolamine
ORNADE 2 FOR CHILDREN: chlorpheniramine, phenylpropanolamine
ORNEX: acetaminophen, phenylpropanolamine
PEDIAQULL: guaifenesin, phenylephrine
PERCOGESIC: acetaminophen, phenyltoloxamine
PERTUSSIN 8-HOUR COUGH FORMULA: dextromethorphan
PERTUSSIN PLUS NIGHT-TIME COLD MEDICINE: acetaminophen,
   chlorpheniramine, dextromethorphan, phenylephrine
PRIVINE: naphazoline
PROPADRINE: phenylpropanolamine
PRUNICODEINE: codeine sulfate, terpin hydrate
PSEUDOEPHEDRINE SYRUP: pseudoephedrine
QUIET-NITE: acetaminophen, chlorpheniramine, dextromethorphan,
   ephedrine
REM: ammonium chloride, dextromethorphan
RHINIDRIN: acetaminophen, phenylpropanolamine, phenyltoloxamine
ROBITUSSIN: guaifenesin
ROBITUSSIN A-C: codeine phosphate, guaifenesin
ROBITUSSIN-CF: dextromethorphan, guaifenesin, phenylpropanolamine
ROMEX: chlorpheniramine, dextromethorphan, guaifenesin, phenylephrine
ROMILAR CF: ammonium chloride, dextromethorphan
ROMILAR CHILDREN'S: dextromethorphan, sodium citrate
ST. JOSEPH COUGH SYRUP FOR CHILDREN: dextromethorphan,
   sodium citrate
ST. JOSEPH DECONGESTANT: oxymetazoline
SILENCE IS GOLDEN: dextromethorphan
SINAREST: acetaminophen, chlorpheniramine, phenylephrine
SINE-AID: acetaminophen, phenylpropanolamine
SINE-OFF: aspirin, chlorpheniramine, phenylpropanolamine
SINE-OFF ONCE-A-DAY NASAL SPRAY: camphor, eucalyptol, menthol,
   xylometazoline

SINEX DECONGESTANT NASAL SPRAY: camphor, eucalyptol, menthol,
   phenylephrine
SINEX LONG-ACTING DECONGESTANT NASAL SPRAY: xylometazoline
SINUTAB TABLETS: acetaminophen, phenylpropanolamine, phenyltoloxamine
SMITH BROTHERS MEDICATED COUGH DROPS: ammonium chloride
SPANTAC: belladonna alkaloids, chlorpheniramine, phenylpropanolamine
SUCRETS COLD DECONGESTANT FORMULA: benzocaine, phenylephrine,
   phenylpropanolamine
SUCRETS COUGH CONTROL FORMULA: dextromethorphan
SUDAFED TABLETS: pseudoephedrine
SUPER ANAHIST NASAL SPRAY: phenylephrine
SUPER ANAHIST TABLETS: acetaminophen, aspirin, phenylpropanolamine,
   phenyltoloxamine
SYMPTOM 1: dextromethorphan
SYMPTOM 2: pseudoephedrine
SYMPTOM 3: brompheniramine
2/G COUGH SYRUP: guaifenesin
TIMED COLD CAPSULES: belladonna alkaloids, chlorpheniramine,
   pheniramine, phenylpropanolamine
TRIAMINIC-DM COUGH FORMULA: dextromethorphan,
   phenylpropanolamine
TRIAMINIC EXPECTORANT: guaifenesin, pheniramine,
   phenylpropanolamine, pyrilamine
TRIAMINICIN NASAL SPRAY: pheniramine, phenylephrine,
   phenylpropanolamine, pyrilamine
TRIAMINICIN TABLETS: aspirin, chlorpheniramine, phenylpropanolamine
TRIAMINICOL DECONGESTANT COUGH SYRUP: ammonium chloride,
   dextromethorphan, pheniramine, phenylpropanolamine, pyrilamine
TRIND-DM SYRUP: acetaminophen, dextromethorphan, guaifenesin,
   phenylephrine
TROCAINE: benzocaine
TUSSAGESIC SUSPENSION: acetaminophen, dextromethorphan,
   pheniramine, phenylpropanolamine, pyrilamine, terpin hydrate
TUSSAGESIC TABLETS: acetaminophen, dextromethorphan, pheniramine,
   phenylpropanolamine, pyrilamine, terpin hydrate
TUSSAR-2: chlorpheniramine, codeine phosphate, guaifenesin, sodium citrate
TUSSAR DM: chlorpheniramine, dextromethorphan, phenylephrine
TUSSAR-SF: chlorpheniramine, codeine phosphate, guaifenesin,
   sodium citrate
TYLENOL: acetaminophen
TYROHIST NASAL SPRAY: phenylephrine, pyrilamine
URSINUS INLAY-TABS: pheniramine, phenylpropanolamine, pyrilamine
VANQUISH: acetaminophen
VAPOSTEAM: camphor, eucalyptus oil, menthol
VICKS COUGH SILENCERS: benzocaine, dextromethorphan
VICKS COUGH SYRUP: dextromethorphan, guaifenesin, sodium citrate
VICKS INHALER: camphor, levodesoxyephedrine, menthol
VICKS VAPORUB: camphor, eucalyptus oil, menthol, turpentine oil
VICKS VATRONOL NOSE DROPS: camphor, ephedrine, eucalyptol, menthol
VICTORS: eucalyptus oil, menthol
VIRO-MED LIQUID: acetaminophen, dextromethorphan, pseudoephedrine,
   sodium citrate
VIRO-MED TABLETS: aspirin, chlorpheniramine, dextromethorphan,
   guaifenesin, pseudoephedrine

# CHAPTER 4

# Influenza—the last infectious plague

**Recognizing the symptoms**
**What you can do to elude flu**
**Treating flu at home**
**Guarding against complications**
**Perfecting a vaccine**
**Should you get a shot?**

"A troublesome cough, with great spitting, also a Catarrh falling down on the palat, throat and nostrils, also accompanied with a feaverish distemper, joyned with heat and thirst, and want of appetite, a spontaneous weariness, and a grievous pain in the back and limbs."

So Thomas Willis, a London physician, described the symptoms of the influenza that struck England in April 1657. Dr. Willis, like most medical experts until the late 19th Century, ascribed the epidemic to a "blast of the stars"; the very name "influenza," according to some scholars, is a contraction of the Italian *influentia coeli*—"celestial influence." So sudden and severe was each epidemic that it seemed logical to attribute the disease to an extraterrestrial event.

Today influenza retains little of its former mystery. Virologists, epidemiologists and medical historians have explained most aspects of the disease and even devised safe annual inoculations that confer temporary immunity to it. Influenza is now known to be an acute, highly contagious respiratory infection caused by a virus slightly larger than most cold viruses. Yet though it is no longer a mystery, flu remains an urgent medical concern. Epidemics occur in many parts of the world each year, and pandemics—extremely severe, global epidemics—erupt at intervals of 10 to 50 years. During an epidemic, as much as 40 per cent of the population may catch flu. Of these, about 1 per cent suffer serious complications, primarily pneumonia.

The death rate from flu and its complications is quite low, about .03 per cent of the United States population during one typical recent outbreak, the 1968-1969 pandemic of Hong Kong flu, but the sheer number of dead is staggering: The pandemic killed 56,000 people in the United States, then recurred the next winter in Europe, killing 30,000 people during an eight-week period in Britain alone. Flu's notoriety stems from its ability to survive and prosper in this fashion when many more deadly diseases have been prevented by universal vaccination or controlled with antibiotics. Influenza is, in fact, the last great infectious plague—and the virus that causes it is one of the most intensively studied infectious agents in all of medicine.

Like the common cold, influenza is strictly a respiratory infection. It affects the nose, throat and chest, not any other parts of the body. The terms "stomach flu" and "intestinal flu" are misnomers. These ailments are caused by gastrointestinal viruses or bacteria. They are unrelated to true influenza and rarely accompany it in adults; on the other hand, children stricken with flu often suffer digestive upsets that are a side effect, not the result of gastrointestinal infection. Particles of a genuine flu virus behave much like cold-virus particles. But the illness itself usually is quite different. Although colds are confined to the nose and throat, classic influenza infects the lower respiratory tract as well and affects the entire body, prostrating its victims for days with fever and widespread muscle aches.

Because the behavior of flu varies so widely that no single symptom distinguishes it from colds, bronchitis, strep throat and other common respiratory infections, it usually is diag-

*Technicians in surgical garb at Wyeth Laboratories in Marietta, Pennsylvania, gather crude flu vaccine — virus-laden fluid — from eggs in which it has been incubated. The virus will be filtered out of the fluid, diluted and refiltered; the process will leave it harmless without eliminating its power to stimulate the production of virus-killing antibodies.*

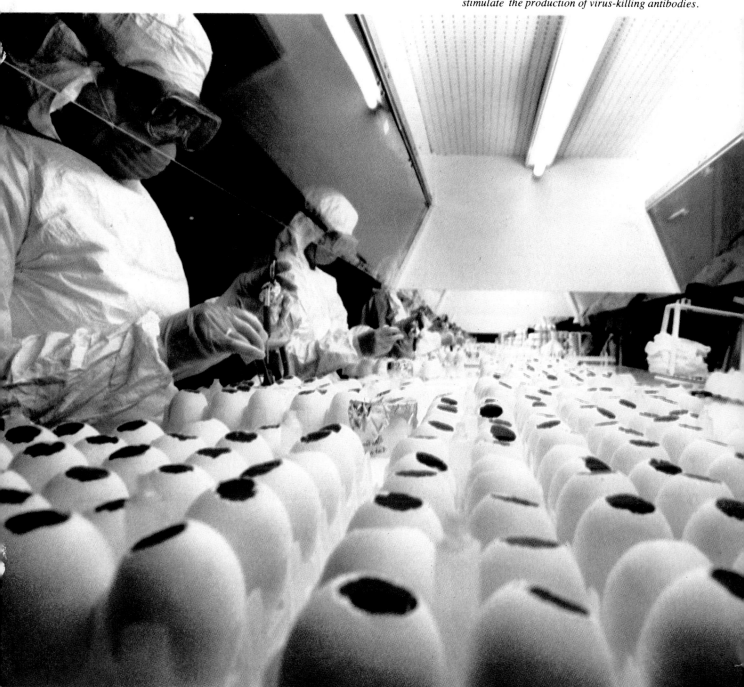

nosed on the basis of several symptoms rather than any one.

● Influenza nearly always starts out with a fever of at least 100° F. Colds rarely are accompanied by fever, except those in children.

● The onset of flu generally is abrupt and severe, in contrast to the slow crescendo of most colds. In one study, 75 per cent of the flu patients were struck suddenly; many could actually pinpoint the exact hour of the attack.

● Flu's constitutional symptoms, such as general weakness, headache, chills and widespread muscle aches, usually overshadow its local cold symptoms, typically sore throat and nasal congestion. Colds, on the other hand, begin with specific local symptoms. Furthermore, in most influenza cases the local symptoms are less severe than those of a full-fledged cold.

● About 90 per cent of flu victims have a dry, hacking cough. Colds are less often accompanied by coughs, and their coughs generally are less painful.

● Sixty per cent of flu victims complain of sore eyes, often accompanied by a burning sensation, redness, watering and sensitivity to light.

● In nearly half of flu cases, patients have a noticeably flushed face and hot, moist skin. Colds seldom cause either of these symptoms in adults.

As the percentage figures indicate, none of these distinctions is absolute. Half the flu cases experience flushing faces, but half do not. That is why distinguishing between a simple cold and the more dangerous influenza requires consideration not only of the symptoms themselves but also of the time at which they appear. A runny nose, for example, usually appears earlier in colds than in flu, as indicated in the comparison chart on page 99.

### Recognizing the symptoms

The course of an individual case of influenza is virtually impossible to predict, but statistical studies have revealed a general pattern. On the first day of illness, a victim's fever rapidly rises to about 101° F. and, in severe cases, as high as 104° F. The fever usually is accompanied by headache, chills and a crushing sense of weariness that confines even a stoic to bed. In most cases, muscle and joint aches develop rapidly—caused, scientists theorize, by by-products that the battling flu-virus particles and white blood cells release into the bloodstream. The "troublesome cough" reported in the 17th Century by Dr. Willis is the most common chest symptom, but in a few flu patients—primarily heavy smokers and those with lung or heart diseases—the cough is a deep, excruciating bark. Even worse, flu often is responsible for a whole list of additional complaints: dizziness, a ticklish throat, loss of appetite, hoarseness, insomnia, slight nausea and—not surprisingly—depression and irritability.

After the first day or two, flu symptoms usually begin to subside, unless complications develop. The fever diminishes each day, usually reaching normal by the fourth day. In a few cases, however, it lasts longer or peaks again on the third or fourth day. As the fever diminishes, constitutional symptoms such as muscle aches gradually abate, leaving in their wake a profound lassitude and predominantly respiratory symptoms. A flu victim generally has a stuffy nose or sore throat for at least three days after fever disappears; the cough persists a few days longer, until the lining of the respiratory tract regenerates. The whole process, from its onset to the return of full health, takes at least a week, occasionally several weeks, and much longer if complications such as bacterial pneumonia ensue.

Children older than 10 years generally suffer the same symptoms as adults, but among younger children the symptoms sometimes differ considerably. Youngsters get flu more often than any other age group, but they usually are afflicted with a mild form of it that may be dismissed as merely a feverish cold. When children do contract full-blown flu, their fever usually exceeds the normal adult range, running higher than 102° F. They frequently suffer diarrhea or vomiting as well as the characteristic flu cough, but they generally escape the muscle aches that plague their elders. Children suffer fewer complications than adults, but those that they do contract can occur suddenly and be quite serious: a dangerous fever (above 104° F.), pneumonia, convulsions and severe croup, which threatens breathing. Any of these may require immediate hospitalization.

# How to tell the difference between flu and a cold

Influenza and the common cold are frequently mistaken for each other because they share many symptoms. A person with a runny nose or a sore throat, for example, may be unsure whether he has come down with a cold or with flu, because these symptoms are associated with both diseases. Yet the distinction is vital, especially for sufferers of chronic heart or lung disease. Such individuals are especially vulnerable to complications of influenza, including pneumonia, pulse irregularities and congestive heart failure. For them, flu is not just a seven-day nuisance; it is a potential killer. They should not try to fight it on their own, but should consult a physician at the first sign of infection.

Fortunately, certain differences between the intensity and duration of cold and flu symptoms can easily be recognized even by the layman. The chart on this page lists 10 symptoms common to both diseases and indicates the prevalence of each symptom on each day of a seven-day spell of cold or flu. To assemble the data for the chart, researchers in Charlottesville, Virginia, monitored the day-to-day symptoms of 139 subjects who had colds and 33 who had Type A flu, using laboratory tests to tell which ailment each subject had.

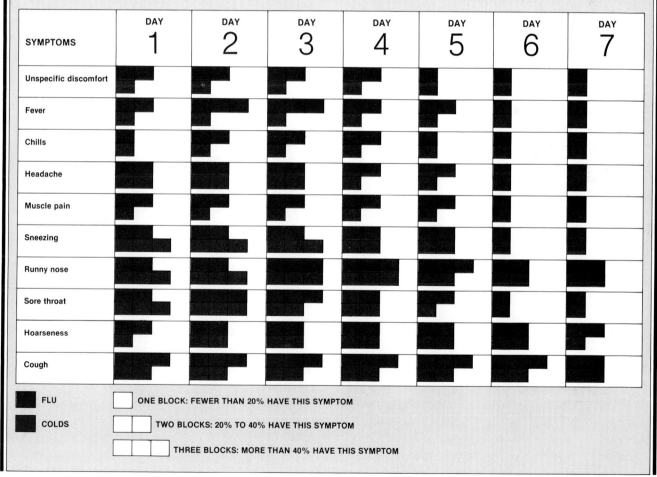

FLU
COLDS
ONE BLOCK: FEWER THAN 20% HAVE THIS SYMPTOM
TWO BLOCKS: 20% TO 40% HAVE THIS SYMPTOM
THREE BLOCKS: MORE THAN 40% HAVE THIS SYMPTOM

*In this chart, colored squares indicate the susceptibility of cold and influenza sufferers to a range of cold and flu symptoms over a seven-day period. In the box for each day, the top half shows the percentage (see key) of flu victims that may expect to have the symptom, while the bottom half indicates the percentage of cold sufferers with the same symptom. For example, on the first day of illness, flu victims are about twice as likely to have fever as are people with colds, but when the illnesses go into their second and third days, fever becomes a more probable symptom of flu by a margin of more than 3 to 1.*

Doctors usually confirm a diagnosis of influenza, not with laboratory tests, but simply by determining whether a flu epidemic is raging in the community. Influenza—unlike colds, which are relatively capricious in their choice of victims—typically races through businesses, schools, churches and other community groups. Isolated cases of flu are so rare that, if you develop flu-like symptoms but find yourself alone in your suffering, you can be reasonably sure that you have something else. By the same token, if you have mild flu symptoms while friends and co-workers around you are also sick, you probably have influenza.

Individual flu cases occur in every month of the year and throughout the world, regardless of climate, but epidemics usually are seasonal. In temperate countries, they are most common in the dead of winter—January through March in the Northern Hemisphere, June through August in the Southern one. Virologists believe that indoor crowding and decreased ventilation during winter play a part in this schedule, as they do in colds. But they also attribute flu's seasonal timing to changes in humidity. Flu viruses thrive in relatively dry air, with a humidity between 15 and 40 per cent—the range maintained by most central-heating systems. Unfortunately, this evidence about epidemics does not mean that individual families can defend themselves against flu by in-

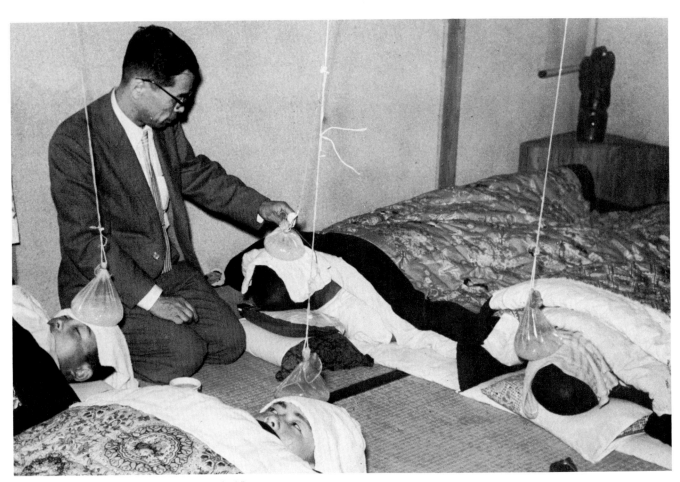

*To soothe a pupil's sudden high fever, typical of flu, a Japanese teacher applies an ice bag hung from the ceiling. During the 1957 Asian flu pandemic, when this picture was made, 10 million people fell victim in 20 weeks, 1.5 million in Japan alone.*

stalling humidifiers. Even in the most humid environment, enough of the hardy virus particles survive to infect people. Although a humidifier will not decrease susceptibility to influenza during the flu season, one set up in a sickroom may ease a flu sufferer's discomfort.

An epidemic usually lasts less than two months, and departs as suddenly as it arrives. In the general population, the infection rate typically is between 10 and 40 per cent; in institutional populations such as boarding schools, the rate sometimes climbs to 75 per cent. But strangely enough, despite this virulence, epidemics move on without striking the entire pool of susceptible people—a result, scientists theorize, of some nonspecific resistance that whole communities develop and share.

**The long search for flu's cause**

Influenza's epidemic nature has been recognized for centuries, but the quest for its cause did not begin in earnest until the end of the 19th Century. The impetus came from the global pandemic of 1889-1890, a cataclysm that spread from Russia across Europe and North America to Australia and India. The decades of ingenious scientific detective work that followed, culminating in the discovery of viruses, revolutionized all of medicine.

At first, a few diehards—among them Charles Creighton, an eminent British scientist—contended that influenza was not even a contagious disease but was caused by a miasma, that is, by noxious, nocturnal vapor. However, most scientists were enthusiastic apostles of Louis Pasteur and Robert Koch, the fathers of modern bacteriology, who in the 1870s and 1880s had stunned the world by demonstrating that microorganisms, transmitted from one person to another, could cause disease. Pasteur, a French chemist, identified the bacteria responsible for several diseases and developed vaccines against chicken cholera, anthrax and rabies. Koch, a German country physician, developed ways to grow pure strains of bacteria in laboratory cultures and to stain bacteria so that they were easily visible under a microscope. Koch also infected healthy animals with laboratory strains, thus proving that the bacteria caused the disease.

Thus, when the 1889 pandemic struck, researchers immediately began looking for the bacteria responsible. Soon Richard Pfeiffer, a German bacteriologist, claimed success, blaming flu on the *Hemophilus influenzae* bacterium—before long simply called Pfeiffer's influenza bacillus. The discovery remained controversial, however, because the new bacterium seldom caused influenza in healthy volunteers—one key test in seeking the cause of a disease.

During the following decades, scientists continued to puzzle over other failures to link disease to specific bacteria. Pasteur himself had realized that the presumed agent of some diseases—rabies, for example—could not be seen under a microscope, and he assumed that the invisible agents were bacteria too small to be seen. But subsequent researchers also found that these mysterious agents, unlike all bacteria known, could not be grown in any of the standard culture media. Stranger still, in 1892 a Russian botanist, Dimitri Ivanovski, unwittingly proved that these agents could pass through a porous porcelain filter that held back all known bacteria. He passed sap from tobacco plants afflicted with a blight called tobacco mosaic disease through a filter, then smeared the filtered fluid on healthy plants—and found that they quickly contracted the disease.

Ivanovski merely assumed that his filters were defective. But in 1898 Martinus Beijerinck, a Dutchman, carried the process one step further and reached a quite different conclusion. Beijerinck, ignorant of Ivanovski's work, again used filtered juice from tobacco plants, but he repeated the experiment again and again with filtered juice from each successive newly infected plant. If the filtered fluid merely contained toxins—chemical poisons that are inanimate by-products of living bacteria, unable to reproduce themselves—this method would so dilute them that they could no longer cause the disease. He found that the agent remained infectious.

Since the filtered juice did not contain bacteria or toxins, Beijerinck reasoned, it must contain something else. And he shrewdly guessed the significant characteristic of his new agent, which would not grow in laboratory cultures. "To reproduce itself," he said of the disease-causing material, it "must be incorporated into the living cytoplasm of the cell, into whose multiplication it is, as it were, passively drawn.'' In the title of his research paper Beijerinck named the mysterious agent *contagium vivum fluidum,* Latin for ''contagious living fluid''; but it soon became known as a virus, the standard Latin label for a biological poison.

Beijerinck's evidence and provocative conjectures established the infant science of virology. But in the first decades of the 20th Century most scientists—deceived, perhaps, by the fact that early virus research involved plants rather than animals—continued to assume that influenza was caused by bacteria. Pfeiffer's *Hemophilus influenzae* remained the prime suspect. Then, in 1918, the world was attacked by the greatest medical catastrophe of the 20th Century—the influenza pandemic of 1918-1919. Historians rank this scourge with such bacterial plagues as the Black Death, which decimated Europe and Asia in the 14th Century. The 1918 flu, variously dubbed Spanish influenza and la grippe, afflicted one fifth of the world's population and killed some 20 million people, nearly three times the number killed in World War I.

## A catastrophic pandemic

The first appearance of the disease was unremarkable: It was a mild but highly contagious flu no different from the types in normal, recurring epidemics. In March 1918 a few small

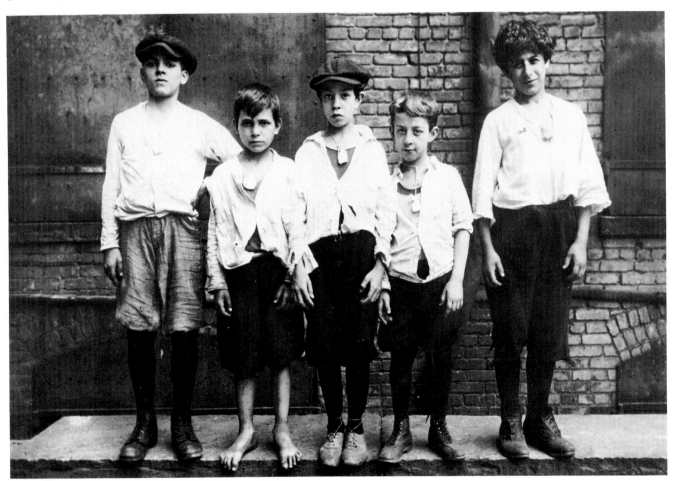

*Camphor bags worn around the necks of these boys reflect the desperate—and futile—measures tried against the great influenza pandemic of 1918-1919 (pages 124-135). Camphor fumes were supposed to kill the flu ''bug,'' but one Montreal doctor had his patients use the potentially lethal substance as a mouthwash and even injected it directly into the bloodstream.*

outbreaks appeared on opposite sides of the world—at Army camps in the United States, where war mobilization was under way, and in China. By April United States troops had carried the disease to France; at the end of the month flu swept into Spain, proving especially potent there; by May, when the contagion finally began to subside in the United States, flu was rampant everywhere on the Continent.

Normal life in some countries came to a virtual standstill. In the space of one month, for example, 53,000 Swiss took to their beds. At midsummer, half of the population of Chungking, in China, was down with flu. The Great War was affected *(pages 124-135)*. So many infantrymen were sick in the German camps along the Marne that General Erich von Lüdendorff despaired of mounting an offensive. Still the disease's deadly potential remained hidden. Most flu victims recovered normally, and medical authorities assumed that the pandemic would soon end.

But in late August, 1918, a new, far more virulent, version of flu suddenly sprang out simultaneously in Boston, in Brest, France, and in Freetown, Sierra Leone—three Atlantic ports actively engaged in the transshipment of men to the European war zone. Within days, the new sickness struck down thousands of soldiers, sailors and civilians, prostrating half of the men in some Army units.

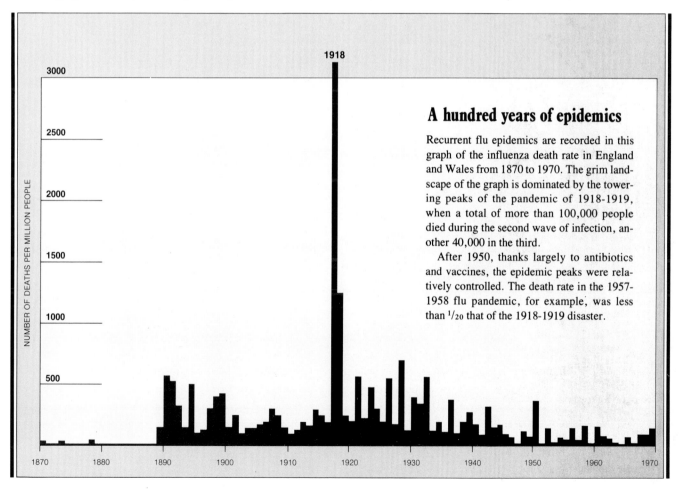

## A hundred years of epidemics

Recurrent flu epidemics are recorded in this graph of the influenza death rate in England and Wales from 1870 to 1970. The grim landscape of the graph is dominated by the towering peaks of the pandemic of 1918-1919, when a total of more than 100,000 people died during the second wave of infection, another 40,000 in the third.

After 1950, thanks largely to antibiotics and vaccines, the epidemic peaks were relatively controlled. The death rate in the 1957-1958 flu pandemic, for example, was less than $1/20$ that of the 1918-1919 disaster.

This second wave of influenza had an alarming tendency to give way to pneumonia, often causing breathing difficulties and death within a day. Treatment was fruitless. "On admission most of the early cases were blue as huckleberries. Most of them died. Nearly all were coughing up liquid blood," one doctor wrote. "We had to stand by helpless except for what temporary relief we could give." Most frightening of all, mortality was highest not among the elderly, the primary victims of most flu epidemics, but among young adults in the prime of life.

Cities from Chicago to Calcutta mobilized for the battle against flu. Theaters and churches were closed by government proclamation and the public was urged to get plenty of bed rest, eat regularly and "beware of persons shaking hands." New York's Commissioner of Health made sneezing and coughing in public places a punishable offense, subject to fine or jailing; he also called for "spitless Sundays" and advised young couples who could not refrain from kissing to do so through handkerchiefs. San Francisco required its citizens to wear face masks in all public buildings—prompting the police to complain that robbers, thus disguised, were more brazen than ever. In every major American metropolis, several hospitals were devoted solely to the care in isolation of flu victims.

Still the toll of sick and dead continued to climb. In the United States alone, 500,000 people died—one person in every 200. In isolated settlements in Alaska, where the Eskimos had had no previous exposure to influenza, casualties soared as high as 100 per cent; in Samoa 25 per cent of the population died.

### Closing in on the cause

When the pandemic ended in the spring of 1919, medical authorities were still unsure what had caused it, why it subsided or how they could prevent another one. Again scientists found Pfeiffer's bacillus in flu victims, but the bacteria still did not always cause flu in healthy volunteers.

Equally baffling, scientists were unable to prove that influenza was caused by a virus. Monkeys, rabbits and other animals were inoculated with filtered throat washings from flu patients, yet they failed to get the disease. Even when, in a risky and heroic experiment, scientists filtered sputum and juices from the lungs of dead flu victims and inoculated human volunteers with the filtrate, illness rarely appeared. (Medical historians theorize that these experiments—which should have worked—failed for one of three reasons: because the dead flu victims were no longer shedding infectious virus particles, because the crude filters available in 1918 held back virus particles along with bacteria, or because the volunteers already had antibodies to the flu.) As late as 1922, Robert Donaldson of St. George's Hospital Medical School in London wrote that "there is not the slightest shred of evidence that the disease is due to a so-called filter-passing virus." The mystery seemed insoluble.

Research on the basic nature of viruses progressed rapidly, however. Soon after the War, virologists turned to animal experiments, which often give conflicting results because of the presence of antibodies or bacterial disease. To surmount these obstacles, scientists devised methods of sustaining live animal tissue in the laboratory—bits of nerve fiber, rabbit cornea, chicken kidney and many other tissues—by bathing them periodically in nutrients. These procedures allowed brief cultivation of animal viruses, but the cultures were constantly plagued by bacterial contamination. To keep ahead of the invading bacteria, researchers in the era before antibiotics had to transfer each culture to a fresh test tube every few days—a process that discouraged the growth of most viruses as well.

The ultimate solution was deceptively simple. In 1928 Dr. Ernest W. Goodpasture and Alice M. Woodruff, two Vanderbilt University scientists, managed—after hundreds of false starts—to grow the fowl-pox virus in nature's own sterile incubators, fertilized chicken eggs. Furthermore, they passed the virus from egg to egg and then returned it to live chickens, conclusively proving the existence of viral disease in animals. They later showed that fertilized eggs—a cheap, convenient laboratory medium—could sustain a variety of human viruses as well.

The final clue in the case of the missing flu virus came not from a physician, but from an astute veterinarian. During the

1918 pandemic J. S. Koen, an Iowa inspector for the U.S. Bureau of Animal Industry, noted a pig disease that resembled Spanish flu. Despite considerable opposition from farmers, who feared that consumers would avoid pork, Koen maintained that the swine disease was connected to human influenza. In 1919 he wrote: "I believe I have as much to support this diagnosis in pigs as the physicians have to support a similar diagnosis in man. The similarity of the epidemic among people and the epidemic among pigs was so close, the reports so frequent, that an outbreak in the family would be followed immediately by an outbreak among the hogs, and vice versa, as to present a most striking coincidence if not suggesting a close relation between the two conditions. It looked like 'flu,' and until proved it was not 'flu,' I shall stand by that diagnosis."

In 1928 Koen's conviction prompted a team of government veterinarians to instill mucus from sick pigs into the noses of healthy ones, which promptly got sick. However, when the veterinarians tried to transmit the disease with filtered mucus, the experiment failed—presumably because the filters were defective. The virus hypothesis remained unproved.

But Richard Shope, a brilliant young pathologist at The Rockefeller Institute for Comparative Pathology in Princeton, New Jersey, was intrigued by the experiments. He visited pig farmers in the Midwest, learning that swine influenza still occurred there every autumn. And in late 1928 Shope repeated the government experiment, this time with the institute's excellent equipment. The filtered fluid consistently produced disease, proving that pig influenza, at least, was caused by a virus.

But the cause of human flu remained elusive. During a 1933 influenza epidemic in England a team of British researchers, Wilson Smith, Christopher Andrewes and P. P. Laidlaw, injected filtrates of human throat washings into various animals. Nothing happened, because (it is now known) the scientists did not try nasal administration, the only practical route for influenza experiments. A few weeks later, however, the virologists learned from the Wellcome Laboratories in London that some ferrets used there in research on canine distemper seemed to have caught flu. Coincidentally, Andrewes himself had just contracted influenza, so Smith inoculated healthy ferrets with filtrate from his sick colleague's throat washings, this time using the nasal route, as Shope had done.

On the day that Andrewes returned to work, the inoculated ferrets developed sneezing, fever and nasal discharge—the classic signs of animal influenza. The British team finally had proved that human flu was caused by a virus. Only later did they learn that their experiment began with a fortuitous fluke: The ferret illness that had initially been reported to them by the Wellcome Laboratories turned out to be canine distemper after all. The final step in the experiment—demonstration that ferret influenza was the same as human influenza—was equally lucky. Three years later, while a researcher was examining an inoculated ferret, the animal sneezed in his face—and the scientist contracted influenza. The proof was complete.

Now research accelerated rapidly. Smith, drawing on Dr. Goodpasture's work, successfully cultivated the flu virus in chicken eggs. Then Wendell M. Stanley, a 31-year-old chemist at The Rockefeller Institute, crystallized a virus—proof that viruses are a transition form between the living and the nonliving. They are inanimate chemical compounds rather than submicroscopic cells, for only chemicals can form crystals. Yet they possess the power to reproduce themselves, as only living things can. British bacteriologist William Elford accurately measured the sizes of different viruses, filtering them through very thin membranes, each graded according to its pore size. And finally, in 1939, German virologists using a new invention, the electron microscope, were able to clearly see the ghostly particles (pages 20-21) that they had studied blindly for so long.

Scientists eventually discovered that human influenza was caused by not just one virus, but three different types of viruses, labeled A, B and C. Type A, the virus that was initially isolated by the British researchers, is the most common type and by far the most important. It is responsible for most flu epidemics and most flu-related deaths in adults. Type B also causes epidemics, though less frequently than A;

it occurs primarily in school-age children. Type C is relatively inconsequential; it erupts only occasionally and then as a very mild infection.

### What the virus does

An influenza virus behaves much like other respiratory viruses. It can produce infections of varying severity, ranging from a "silent" infection, with no symptoms at all, to a sudden and severe disease. The extent of the infection depends primarily on the victim's own supply of antibodies, germ-killing substances specifically compounded to combat each flu strain. If you are lucky enough to pass through a flu epidemic without getting sick, you may have already had antibodies quite similar to those that are effective against the prevalent virus. Even if you merely feel vaguely out of sorts without actually getting sick, your infection will trigger antibody production that can give you years of immunity to that particular virus. In fact, antibodies provide such a good record of a person's exposure to flu that scientists have dated 19th and early-20th Century epidemics and identified the viruses involved by analyzing the antibodies in the blood of people of different age groups.

Influenza spreads the same way colds do: Virus particles hitch a ride aboard droplets blown into the air by the coughs and sneezes of a sufferer. However, influenza-carrying droplets are much more infectious than those bearing cold viruses. Most researchers believe that flu is carried not only in relatively large droplets like those that transport cold viruses, but also in tiny droplets—as small as $1/25,000$ inch in diameter, a fraction of the size of the smallest cold-laden droplet. This microscopic mist can remain airborne and infectious for an hour or more, floating in theaters, offices, restaurants and any other closed space. Even a tightly fitting surgical mask does not filter out such minuscule droplets, although it can block large ones.

After the respiratory tract is infected, an incubation period follows before a victim suddenly feels sick. The duration of incubation depends on the virus dosage; it ranges between one and four days, averaging about two. During this period, as in the corresponding stage of a cold, virus particles invade

## How the virus takes hold

An influenza infection is a drama of subversion played out at the microscopic level of the cell. A virus particle enters the respiratory system, insinuates its way into a healthy cell and makes it produce copies of the virus. After about six hours, hundreds of new flu particles launch themselves into the respiratory channels.

A particle of influenza A—the commonest, most severe type—has several structural features to help it do its work. Up to 1,000 spikes of protein compounds grow from its surface. There are two kinds of compound. One, hemagglutinin, matches a protein on the host cell's surface, as a key matches a lock, opening the cell for invasion. The other kind of spike, neuraminidase, clears the virus surface of a substance that otherwise makes it stick to other particles, producing a clump too big to squeeze into a cell.

Another feature unique to the flu virus—one that helps make it a formidable opponent—lies in the genetic material that controls its reproduction. In the flu virus the genes consist of eight separate pieces (in a common-cold virus the genetic material is one continuous strand). Each time a flu-virus particle reproduces itself, the eight new genes must form the correct pattern. Occasionally a mutation occurs, producing genes with a slightly different molecular makeup. If this strain prospers, a new variety of virus arises: not a totally different, pandemic-causing breed, but one distinct enough to resist vaccines that protected against its forebears.

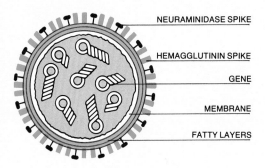

NEURAMINIDASE SPIKE

HEMAGGLUTININ SPIKE

GENE

MEMBRANE

FATTY LAYERS

**THE INGREDIENTS OF INFLUENZA**
*Each influenza particle is designed to enter a human cell, where it reproduces itself. The hemagglutinin and neuraminidase spikes, which work together to get the virus inside a body cell, are anchored in two fatty layers. These layers cover a membrane that encloses the genes, or hereditary material.*

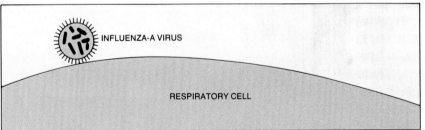

**INFECTION: ATTACHMENT TO A CELL**
*A particle of influenza-A virus, one of hundreds that may be inhaled in a single airborne droplet, approaches a cell of the respiratory system. The hemagglutinin spikes find a vulnerable spot on the cell surface, and a chemical bond immediately forms between host and invader.*

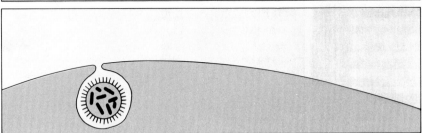

**FIRST HOUR: PENETRATION**
*About 30 minutes after the virus particle becomes attached, the cell engulfs it. Toward the end of this stage, the cell surface will close over the virus particle.*

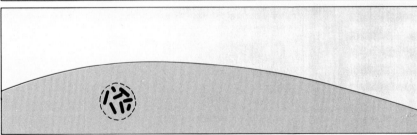

**SECOND HOUR: UNCOATING**
*Chemical activators, or enzymes, in the cell dissolve the fatty layers and membrane enclosing the virus particle. The heredity-controlling material—the genes—of the virus are released inside the cell to take over the cell's own reproductive mechanisms.*

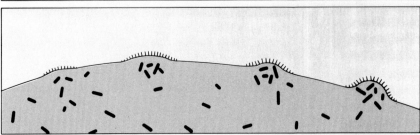

**FIFTH HOUR: BUDDING**
*The virus genes force the cell to manufacture duplicates of themselves. These newly made virus genes migrate to the edge of the cell. There they arrange themselves in bundles, each having eight genes identical to the parent's. New spikes begin poking out in patches all around the cell surface.*

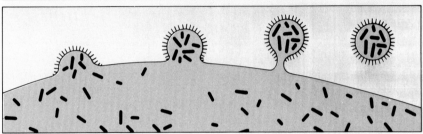

**SIXTH HOUR: RELEASE**
*As many as 1,000 flu particles bud forth before the host cell is destroyed by the infection. As the process repeats itself and more host cells die, the body begins to feel the first effects of the influenza attack.*

*How new (or apparently new) strains of influenza arise is unsettled, but two possible explanations are diagramed on these pages. According to one theory (below), a virus (red) becomes so prevalent in humans that it cannot spread much further; it then infects animals, such as pigs (pink). Generations later, when millions of people lack antibodies to fight it, it reattacks humans.*

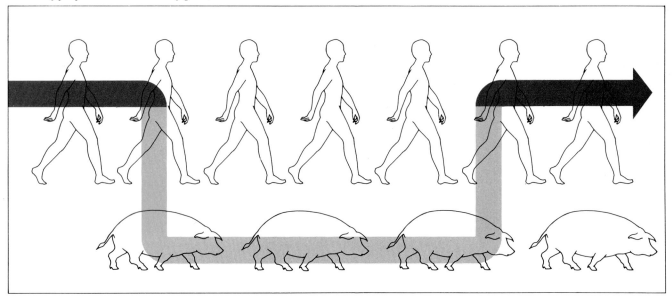

the mucous membrane cells of the nose, the throat and the bronchial tubes, shed their protective envelopes, and commandeer cell machinery, forcing the cells to produce more virus particles. In a matter of five or six hours, the viral offspring—as many as 1,000 particles in each infected cell—begin to bud out from the cell's wall and go forth as infectious legions to repeat the destructive process. Quite different from cold viruses, however, are the component parts of the influenza virus.

The surface of an influenza virus bristles like a medieval mace with two dangerous sorts of protein spikes. (The spikes are also, significantly, the components that trigger a flu victim's production of antibodies during recovery from infection.) One type of spike, consisting of a substance called neuraminidase, chemically dissolves the blanket of mucus that protects the mucous membrane, laying bare the living cell. The other, hemagglutinin, glues the virus to a receptor on the surface of the host cell. The next step in the process is somewhat mysterious: Hemagglutinin somehow stimulates the host cell to wrap itself around the virus particle. Once it is trapped, the virus can begin forcing the cell to manufacture duplicate viruses. When this process is complete, neuramini-

dase dissolves the bond between the new virus particles and the cell, allowing the new particles to float away and repeat the process *(pages 106-107).*

## A viral chameleon

The primary reason that the flu virus is such a formidable agent lies in the virus core, which controls the virus's heredity and determines its characteristics and behavior. In most cold viruses, and in most living cells as well, the hereditary core is a continuous strand of compounds whose sequence never changes. Such conventional packages reproduce copies of themselves forever, with little likelihood of an accidental variation along the way; as a result, descendants of a common-cold agent such as the rhino virus are nearly always carbon copies of their ancestors in every respect: size, shape, disease-causing potential and so on.

The hereditary material of the flu virus, by contrast, consists of eight separate fragments—a less stable arrangement that allows more frequent changes in offspring, principally in the chemical composition of the two surface proteins, neuraminidase and hemagglutinin. New variants do not match antibodies that are keyed to the surface spikes of the

*Differing slightly from the theory described at left, another explanation for shifts in flu strains also depends on animal hosts (below). It assumes that, by chance, an animal is infected simultaneously by a human flu virus (red) and by a strain exclusive to animals (blue). The strains merge, producing a hybrid flu (purple) against which humans have no antibody protection.*

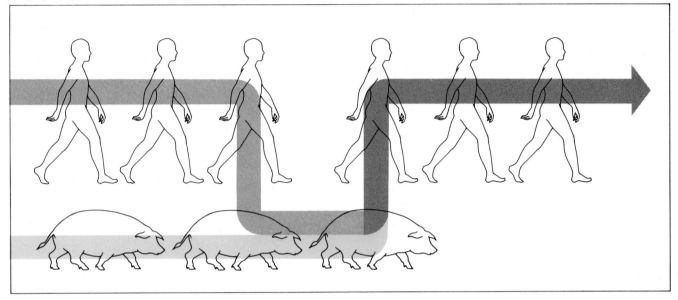

old virus, so the new viruses tend to meet less immune resistance than the previous strain and gradually supersede it. Because an individual's ability to resist reinfection by a particular flu virus is highest when his antibodies already are keyed to that virus, the degree of change in the new variant will largely determine its severity in the individual and in the community. Modest changes, known to virologists as "drifts," cause minor epidemics, since existing antibodies react fairly well against viruses that resemble the one they originally were keyed to. But major changes, or "shifts," produce viruses foreign to the existing store of antibodies and usually cause severe epidemics and pandemics.

Scientists believe that drift is the result of randomly produced new variations in individual flu viruses, which gradually are selected out by nature over older viruses. Unfortunately, human antibodies are not updated in the same way. A person's encounter with each new, slightly different variant primarily triggers antibodies from his first encounter with a related strain. In subsequent encounters, antibodies aimed specifically at the drifted strain will be recalled, but in much smaller amounts. Ordinarily this defense system works fairly well, because antibodies to one strain usually can defeat related ones. But when repeated drift gradually creates a virus quite different from the original, the old antibodies are useless and the hapless victim contracts the new strain of flu. Within the population as a whole, an accumulation of such drifts finds most people completely unprepared and causes a good-sized epidemic.

Virologists once believed that a shift was merely the product of a series of drifts, but modern analytic techniques have revealed that new virus subtypes are so radically different from their predecessors that shift and drift probably are completely different phenomena. Two major theories have been proposed to explain the dynamics of flu viruses' shift, and the truth may combine both of them.

One major theory ascribes shifts to the recirculation of old flu subtypes that have been dormant for decades. According to this hypothesis, as more and more of the population develops antibodies to a particular flu strain, the virus may go into storage—perhaps in the arctic tundra or in animals *(left)*. Barnyard storage is a distinct possibility, because pigs, horses, ducks and chickens all suffer from influenza strains quite similar to human ones. The virus could reside in animals either actively, as animal influenza, or in a latent state that causes no active disease. After a time, when a generation of humans appears lacking antibodies against that virus, the stored virus presumably returns with new vigor and rapidly reemerges as the dominant flu strain.

The second theory also draws on the idea of animal storage. But in this scenario, crossbreeding may take place between two strains of the same virus type, one normally native to animals, the other to humans *(page 109)*. Such an encounter between two flu viruses can take place in a human host, but it is most likely in a more hospitable animal, particularly wild birds, which harbor a wide variety of flu strains. If two different flu viruses simultaneously infect the same cell, their fragmented bits of hereditary material are likely to become shuffled. The progeny of this marriage may possess characteristics of both parents—the surface spikes of an avian strain, perhaps, and the ability to infect human cells. Such a radical shift would find a world of undefended individuals—and cause a pandemic.

Whatever the true explanation of drift and shift may be, they take place within a predictable time period. Minor viral variants, or drifts, occur every two or three years on the average; their infections tend to be of a mild epidemic magnitude in the first year, milder still in the second and third. Such drift cycles rarely make newspaper headlines. Major shifts take place at irregular intervals, anywhere from 10 to 50 years apart. The flu pandemic of 1918-1919 was caused by a shift. So, presumably, were some 30 other pandemics that have been charted by medical historians from health records going back as far as 1510.

## What you can do to elude flu

Whether by drift or by shift, you are likely at one time or another to have a bout of flu. How nasty a bout it is will depend primarily upon your stock of antibodies, but also on your general state of health, the dose of influenza virus that comes your way and several other factors. The precautions against catching flu are similar to the ones that help you minimize infection by colds, with one additional but uncertain weapon—flu vaccination, which is recommended for certain segments of the population. But because you are at serious risk from flu only during an epidemic, it is easier to put your best efforts into observing the precautions for this relatively short period.

Unfortunately, the virulence and wide dispersal of airborne flu particles require safeguards more sweeping than those for colds—so sweeping, in fact, that some people choose to take their chances with influenza rather than forgo all social life for the duration of each epidemic. For those at risk from flu's life-threatening complications, however—people with heart or lung ailments, and those older than 65—and for people who ordinarily have a bad time with flu, the precautions are sensible.

The biggest problem in guarding against the flu is recognizing the onset of an epidemic. News reports and flu alerts declared by public health authorities both are belated indicators, because they announce the presence of an epidemic only when its toll already is high. Word-of-mouth evidence comes earlier and is generally quite reliable. As soon as friends, neighbors, school children or co-workers begin taking sick, it is time to institute your own flu precautions.

Avoid crowds whenever possible during a flu outbreak. That means staying out of theaters, sports arenas and convention halls, and passing up parties. Avoid public transportation when you can; if the distance to be covered is a comfortable walk, there is no sense in sharing a limited air space with virus-shedding flu victims. If you find yourself in the company of a sneezer, a cougher or someone you know has flu, keep your distance.

If someone in your household is a flu victim, your own chances of escaping the disease are not good. Nonetheless, if you follow the rules for avoiding a cold infection that are given in Chapter 2 and observe a few additional ones, you do have a fighting chance.

Isolate the flu sufferer in a separate bedroom. Ideally, set aside a separate bathroom; if that is not possible, at least keep a separate towel and a separate glass reserved for the patient at the bathroom washbasin. (There is no need to segregate the patient's dishes and eating implements, however; the soap and water of ordinary dishwashing will wash away virus particles.) Beware of using the same telephone, another po-

*Circulatory ailments (red) cause more flu-related deaths than any other complication. Among the pneumonias (blue), those involving staphylococcus bacteria or the flu virus are worst because they are resistant to drugs. Other causes of death (green) include diabetes, tuberculosis, asthma, Reye's syndrome (pages 113-115) and Guillain-Barré syndrome (page 121).*

# Who dies of flu and why

That influenza can kill has been recognized for centuries, but until recently no one knew how deadly it could be. The reason is simple: When a victim dies, he dies not from flu but from its complications, such as pneumonia or congestive heart failure, and physicians ascribe death to the complication rather than to flu itself. Thus the routine vital statistics compiled by governments around the world do not record influenza's true mortality rate. The missing statistics are of more than academic interest; they could be used to help identify the individuals who run the greatest risk from flu, and suggest ways of protecting them.

To solve this problem, statisticians have devised an indicator that is tailored to flu's peculiarities. They compare the overall death rate in years of flu epidemics with the overall rate in years when there are no epidemics. The difference between these figures is the "excess" mortality, presumably linked to influenza. Such analyses can be made for various age groups *(right, bottom)*, to find out who dies during a flu year, and for various complications, to find out why they die.

Studies of excess mortality have brought some surprises. The most striking revelation is found in the age breakdown of flu deaths. The general pattern is quite consistent, and it contradicts long-held assumptions. Children, who often contract flu and were thought to be greatly endangered by it, rarely succumb to it. The elderly are the ones who face serious risk. Three quarters of those who die from flu are over 65 years of age.

The statistics on excess mortality have also revealed that pneumonia, which was once considered the major cause of flu-related fatalities, is only one of several leading causes. Epidemiologists now believe that a major flu epidemic may precipitate more deaths from heart attack and from other heart diseases than from pneumonia. The stress of contracting flu can bring on a fatal episode, but because heart diseases often strike so suddenly that the victim is dead before flu is diagnosed, such deaths had not previously been ascribed to influenza.

Vulnerability to such flu-related diseases depends to a great extent on an individual's general health. A 1957 study in Sheffield, England, found that the death rate among people who were hospitalized with flu complications but were otherwise in good health was 19 per cent. Among hospitalized flu victims who also suffered from lung diseases such as emphysema, the death rate was 25 per cent. Among flu patients who had heart ailments the death rate was 42 per cent.

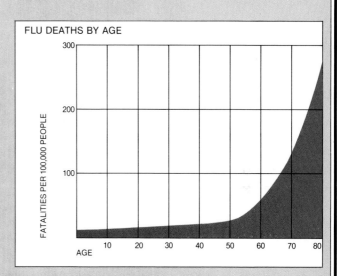

FLU DEATHS BY AGE

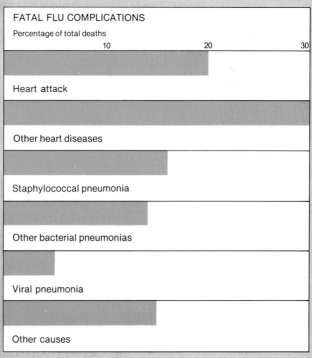

FATAL FLU COMPLICATIONS

Percentage of total deaths

Heart attack

Other heart diseases

Staphylococcal pneumonia

Other bacterial pneumonias

Viral pneumonia

Other causes

*How age affects the danger of influenza is traced in this chart, based on several English and U.S. studies. The high death rate for the elderly had long been known, but not the relatively low death rate for children. Youngsters are seriously endangered by many other respiratory diseases, but not by influenza.*

tent transmitter of viruses, immediately after a flu patient; an hour or two later, after any exhaled moisture has dried, the phone is safe because flu particles are harmless after they have dried.

Wash your hands frequently, especially while caring for someone in the early stages of sickness, when virus shedding is greatest; shedding usually stops after three or four days of illness. Be scrupulous about not rubbing your eyes and nose. Be kind to your body—get plenty of sleep and nutritious food. Some researchers believe that fatigue and psychological stress render people more susceptible to flu—one of the reasons that influenza epidemics are particularly severe at military bases, where recruits are subjected to rigorous training and strict discipline. If you have a temporary or chronic illness, coddle yourself more than you normally would.

### Treating flu at home

If, after such precautions, you still get sick, do not try to maintain your normal routine. Even if you feel only mildly indisposed, you are shedding infectious material and will do everyone a favor if you stay home for the first few days.

Check your temperature two or three times a day—preferably morning, noon and evening, at the same hours each day—and keep a log of the times and readings. The log allows you to chart the course of the disease and spot the warning signs of any complications. If an adult's temperature runs above normal for more than three days, if it reverts to near normal and then soars several days later, or if it goes above 102°, call a physician; high or prolonged fever could indicate a secondary infection that requires professional care. If you have a temperature over 105°, breathing difficulty, severe chest pain or rust-colored mucus, get medical attention immediately—from an emergency room if your personal doctor is unavailable.

The treatment of flu symptoms begins with complete, uncompromising bed rest, which ensures that all available energies are directed toward fighting the infection. If the fever causes great discomfort, headaches or muscle aches, control it with aspirin or an aspirin substitute for an adult, a substitute alone for children. If normal doses of painkiller do not help,

call a physician. To counteract the dehydration brought on by fever, drink lots of fluids, as much as eight ounces of hot or warm nonalcoholic beverages every two hours; a child should drink every 30 minutes, since smaller amounts are consumed. Alcoholic beverages are dangerous; they interact with aspirin and aggravate dehydration.

Smoking should be stopped altogether. Flu viruses strip away layers of cells from the respiratory tract, exposing wounded tissue that smoking irritates easily. If the cough and nasal congestion are pronounced, try the over-the-counter cold preparations described in Chapter 3, with one important exception: A productive cough—one that is bringing up mucus—should not be treated with cough suppressants, because such a cough is essential to keep fluid and bacteria out of the lungs.

Perhaps the best treatment of all for mild flu is psychological. Depression often accompanies the first few days of illness, particularly in people who hate to abandon their normal routine. A cheerful sickroom, soft lighting that will not hurt irritated eyes, and nutritious food treats and beverages help the time pass more comfortably. If sweating is profuse, a cool wipe-down with water or alcohol, followed by fresh bedclothes and linens, gives a tremendous lift to depressed spirits.

Gradual resumption of normal activities should begin no sooner than one full day after body temperature has returned to normal. That period will give you time to be sure that the favorable signs are genuine. Too often people who leap up from their beds prematurely suffer a relapse later, or contract a serious bacterial infection. Even when you are circumspect in the use of your reduced energies after flu, do not be surprised if you need extra sleep and rest for a few weeks. If you are accustomed to exercising strenuously, return to your normal routine gradually, since your lungs may have suffered some temporary damage.

### Guarding against complications

The great majority of flu victims recover uneventfully and fully. Only about 1 per cent develop complications that require hospitalization. But those rare complications can be

# A close call with a fast-moving child killer

Reye's syndrome is a mysterious children's disease that has been linked to the use of aspirin to treat influenza. Named after Dr. Ralph Reye, the pathologist who described it in 1963, the disease follows a viral infection and may strike one child in 100,000.

Like two-year-old Cissy Smith *(below),* the typical victim is affected while recovering from flu. Symptoms appear in rapid succession: vomiting and listlessness, then irritability, delirium, disturbed breathing, stiffness and coma. The liver enlarges, and seems to trigger an accumulation of fluid in the brain, causing pressure and, ultimately, brain damage or death. No cause or cure has been found, but early diagnosis and intensive care have improved the survival rate. Today, more than three quarters of the victims recover. Although aspirin has not been proved a cause, parents are now cautioned against using it for most children's flu.

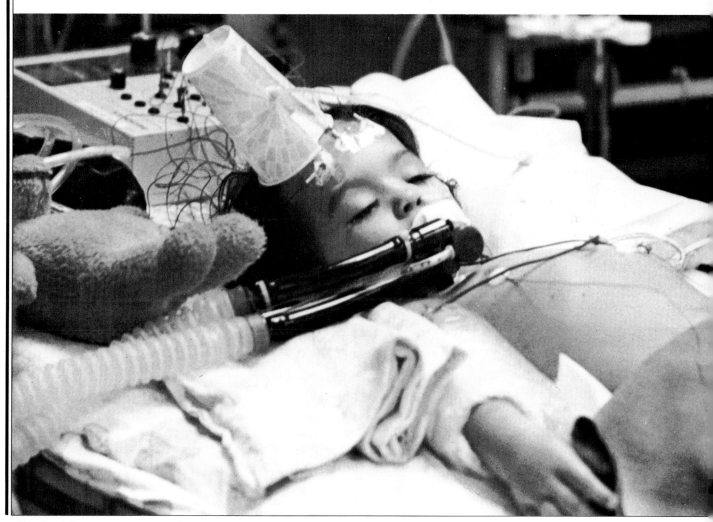

*Cissy Smith lies comatose, arms stiffly extended in the posture typical of Reye's syndrome. In her third day at the intensive care unit of Oakland, California's Children's Hospital, respirator tubes control her breathing, an electroencephalograph (top left) takes brain-wave readings and, under a protective paper cup, a probe inserted through her skull monitors brain pressure.*

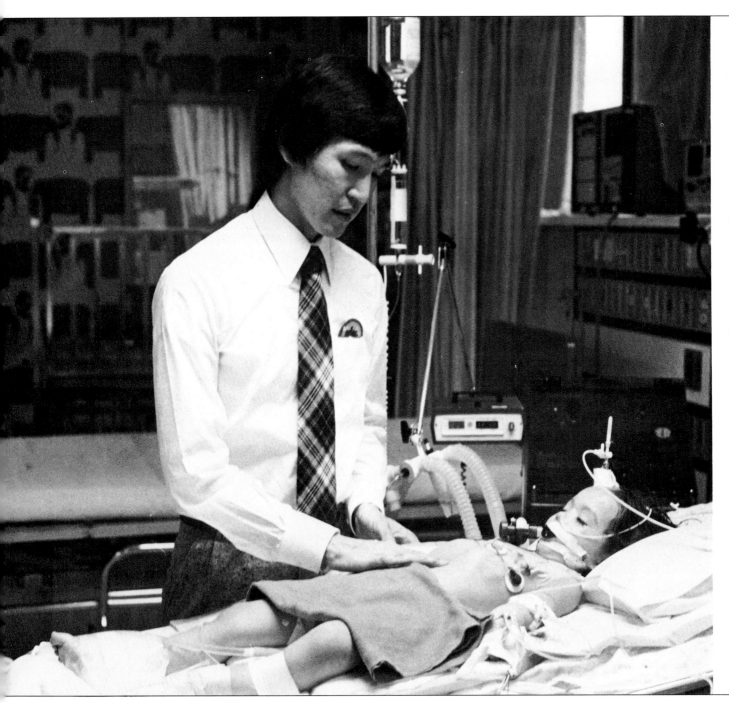

*On the second day of treatment, Dr. Brian Aoki examines the
unconscious child for signs of a change in the size of her liver. The
life-support devices surrounding doctor and patient include a
thermal blanket and mattress, intravenous lines for nutrients and
drugs (behind the doctor), and a bladder catheter.*

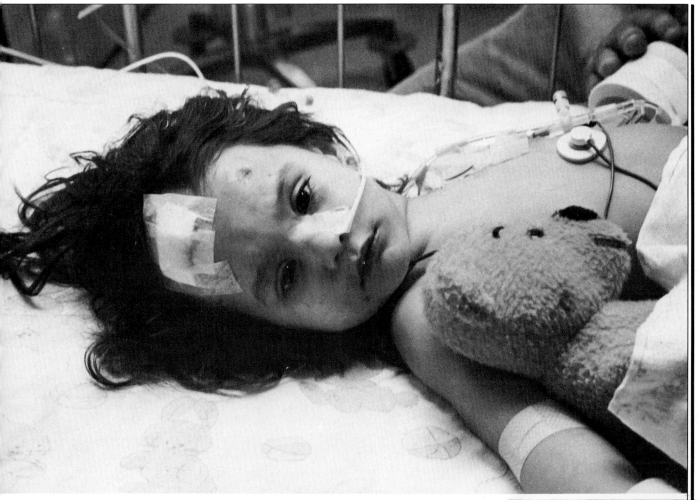

Seven days after entering the hospital, a dazed Cissy regains
consciousness (above) and says a few words. Having found
no evidence of permanent brain or liver damage, the doctors have
begun to remove Cissy's electrodes and monitors, leaving
her with a patchwork of temporary scars and bandages. Less than
a week after this photograph was taken, the toddler was ready
to go home, a record for Reye's syndrome patients. She went on
to a full and vigorous recovery: Four months later she was
riding her tricycle (right) while her brother watched.

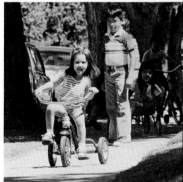

## Viral pneumonia: mysteries of a killer

The deadliest complication of influenza is viral pneumonia, which results when the virus causing influenza spreads into the lungs. In ordinary years, it is blamed for 5 per cent of all influenza-associated deaths; in years of influenza pandemics, the figure soars to 12 per cent.

Viral pneumonia is so dangerous because, unlike the types of pneumonia caused by bacteria, it cannot be cured with antibiotics. However, modern methods of treatment, combined with accurate, speedy diagnosis that helps to catch the disease in its early stages, can change the bleak picture. The treatments are essentially supportive—oxygen to aid the heart, suction to clear away mucus, intravenous feeding to maintain strength, and respirators to provide breathing assistance—but they seem to be effective if begun early enough. One small study followed the course of 11 pneumonia sufferers—all but one past middle age—during the 1976 epidemic of influenza in Seattle. Six of them died. The five who survived were sent to the hospital much sooner and were put on mechanical respirators sooner.

Even so, the overall fatality rates for flu-related viral pneumonia remain tragically high. Only about a quarter of all victims survive, a record that has not improved greatly in decades. As the authors of the Seattle study, Drs. Richard H. Winterbauer, W. Richard Ludwig and Samuel P. Hammar, somberly observed, the disease is "a catastrophic illness with rare survivors."

Still in the future are antiviral drugs that can stop viral pneumonia the way antibiotics cure bacterial pneumonia; several are under intensive study. Improved methods for administering such drugs may also help. In Texas, researchers from the Baylor College of Medicine tested an aerosol mist *(page 150)* that could allow physicians to deliver concentrated drugs directly to the lungs. But Dr. Robert Couch, director of the Influenza Research Center there, cautioned that, for the present, the simplest and most promising treatment for viral pneumonia is prevention of influenza itself by more effective vaccines and more widespread immunization.

serious. Bacterial pneumonia, an inflammation of the lung tissue by any of several bacteria, is the most common complication. Like flu, it is associated with high fever, chills, chest pain and constitutional malaise. When coming in on the coattails of flu, it usually reveals itself as a rebound or additional boost in temperature—occasionally up to a dangerously high 105° or 106° F. The thin, watery mucus that accompanies the cough of influenza turns to a copious, thick, yellow or greenish material, sometimes rust-colored by blood. Breathing becomes shallow and difficult and, in consequence, it speeds up; so does the pulse rate. In critical cases cyanosis—a faint blue tinge under the fingernails, on the lips, on the tips of the ears or over the cheekbones, which is a sign of insufficient oxygen—may be noticeable.

Bacterial pneumonia often is caused by mucus that seeps down into the lungs. Seepage can occur, for example, if influenza viruses severely damage the cilia lining parts of the respiratory tract; the cilia, which normally move mucus into the gastrointestinal tract, may no longer be able to dispose of mucus safely. The mucus contains bacteria such as *Hemophilus influenzae,* streptococcus and staphylococcus. They ordinarily are quite harmless, but when large numbers of such bacteria multiply in the normally sterile reaches of the lower respiratory tract, they become highly destructive. Before the age of antibiotics, such invaders almost invariably caused fatal infections. Even today, with antibiotics that can cure bacterial pneumonia, the disease kills about 25 per cent of those hospitalized with it.

Viral pneumonia *(page 116),* a rarer lung infection caused by the influenza virus itself, offers a still bleaker prognosis. This disease usually behaves like an extraordinarily vicious influenza, with rapid onset, an unrelenting cough and soaring fever; most cases of viral pneumonia end in death from respiratory or cardiac collapse.

Other secondary illnesses, while less serious, present a greater range of symptoms and dangers. Bronchitis is normally part of flu; the term merely indicates an inflammation of the bronchial tubes, which lead from the windpipe to the lungs. Occasionally a bacterial infection aggravates this condition. Milder than pneumonia, bacterial bronchitis nonetheless represents an escalation in the patient's general state of respiratory distress and requires medical attention; it can develop into pneumonia. A pronounced dry, short cough gradually develops into a moist-sounding cough as mucus accumulates and begins to loosen in the bronchial passages. Often, the wheezing of simple breathing becomes audible across a room.

Sinusitis, an inflammation of the mucous membrane that lines the sinus cavities, often is caused by interference in the normal drainage of the sinuses. The condition arises either when the viral infection spreads to the sinuses or when mucus fails to drain normally through the sinus canals, allowing time for bacteria in the mucus to infect the sinuses. If the infection is left untended for weeks, it may become chronic. Severe cases are commonly treated with decongestants and antibiotics; if drugs do not help, a doctor must draw off the pus-filled mucus.

Otitis media, an infection of the middle ear, is caused by inflammation and blockage of the narrow Eustachian tubes, which run from the ears to the throat. Earache, fever and temporarily impaired hearing are the classic signs. Because of the small diameter of children's Eustachian tubes, youngsters are especially susceptible to otitis media. Failure to treat earaches can result in permanent loss of hearing or an infection of nearby organs, including the brain. Fortunately, antibiotics and decongestants usually control otitis media within a few days.

Cardiac complications, ranging from transitory changes in heartbeat to heart attack or congestive heart failure, are less common but extremely serious. They occur primarily in people with a history of heart or lung trouble. Such persons should be under their physician's care from the first sign of influenza, however mild.

Unusual risks from flu may face one special class of individuals: pregnant women. The effect on them of influenza Type A, the classic influenza of epidemics, is still somewhat uncertain. Healthy pregnant women and their babies do not normally suffer special adverse effects from influenza, but there is some statistical evidence that pregnant women who contract influenza have a higher risk of miscarriage and that their babies have a slightly higher rate of birth defects. During the shifts in 1918 and 1957, mortality among pregnant women increased as well—but this hazard has not been documented in other epidemics. A pregnant woman should seek a physician's advice if she catches influenza.

Type B influenza seldom afflicts adults. In children, however, it does have a relationship with Reye's syndrome *(pages 113-115)*, a mysterious, swift-moving disorder, first identified in 1963, that can profoundly disrupt liver and brain function. In the United States the syndrome currently occurs in one case out of 20,000 Type B influenza cases reported. Frequently fatal in the past, owing partly to the difficulty doctors had in diagnosing the unfamiliar disease, Reye's syndrome is now better known and somewhat less dangerous but still a serious hazard. Its fatality rate has dropped from 42 per cent to 21 per cent in recent years.

**Perfecting a vaccine**

Because influenza can be so dangerous to some people, efforts were begun soon after the identification of the influenza virus to create an effective vaccine against it. Researchers soon discovered that the many strains of flu made successful flu vaccinations considerably more difficult to achieve than in the case of other infectious diseases.

Vaccination is a technique for inducing immunity to a viral disease by artificially stimulating a person's production of antibodies against a specific virus. Doctors inoculate the patient with a virus that has been modified to limit its ability to reproduce but is still capable of stimulating production of antibodies.

The principal flu vaccine used today, inactivated (often called "killed") virus vaccine, is prepared by growing a human flu virus in fertilized chicken eggs, then inactivating it with formalin, a formaldehyde solution. The formalin chemically bonds to the hemagglutinin and neuraminidase spikes on the surface of each virus particle, in effect clogging them so that they can no longer infect human cells. The clogged spikes, however, still retain their power to trigger normal antibody response, thus conferring immunity to the disease.

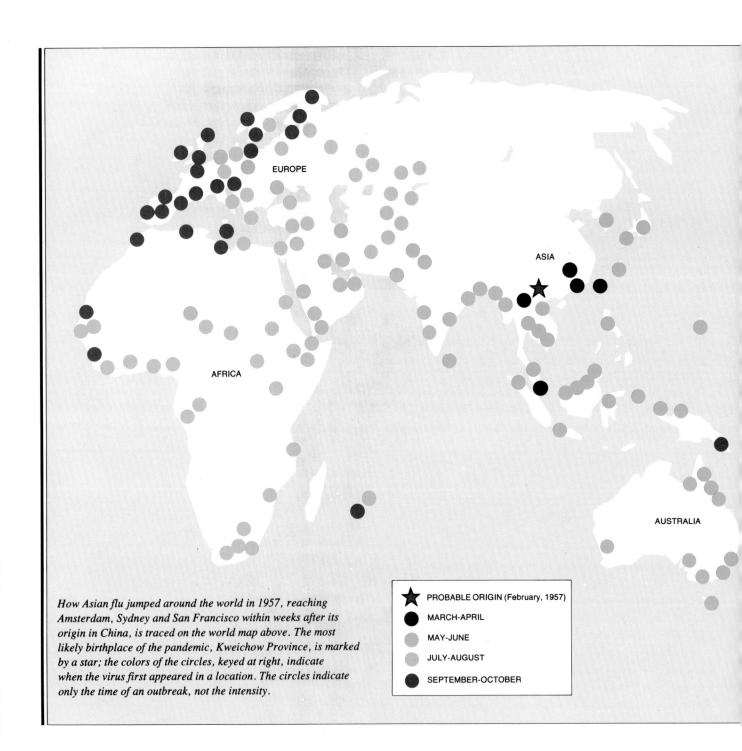

EUROPE

ASIA

AFRICA

AUSTRALIA

How Asian flu jumped around the world in 1957, reaching
Amsterdam, Sydney and San Francisco within weeks after its
origin in China, is traced on the world map above. The most
likely birthplace of the pandemic, Kweichow Province, is marked
by a star; the colors of the circles, keyed at right, indicate
when the virus first appeared in a location. The circles indicate
only the time of an outbreak, not the intensity.

★ PROBABLE ORIGIN (February, 1957)

● MARCH-APRIL

● MAY-JUNE

● JULY-AUGUST

● SEPTEMBER-OCTOBER

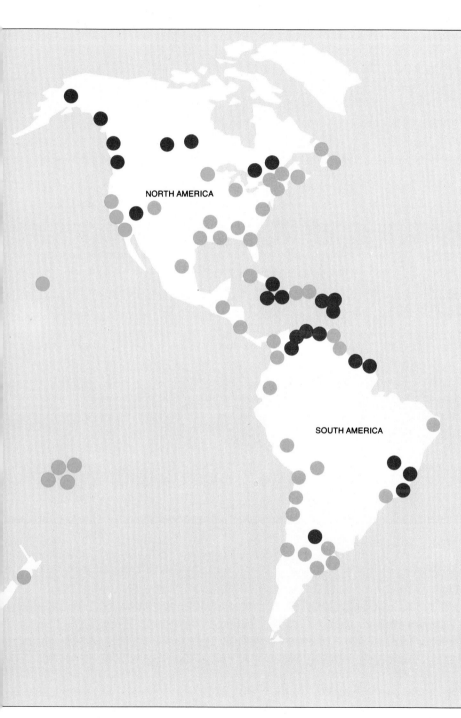

## Tracking a pandemic around the globe

Early in 1957, in southern China, a new and potent strain of Type A influenza appeared. Six months later it had leaped all around the globe. It was the most severe pandemic since the disaster of 1918-1919.

But far fewer people died in 1957 than in the earlier pandemic, which had taken the world by surprise. Even before the so-called Asian flu left the Far East, a worldwide network of scientists was mobilized. Researchers at about 30 laboratories identified the new strain and traced local patterns of infection. This information was rushed to World Health Organization centers in London and Montgomery, Alabama. There epidemiologists mapped the course of the disease.

In the United States, the Surgeon General announced that the medical community was "ahead of an impending epidemic of influenza" for the first time in history. Staying ahead had become essential, for fast air and sea travel spread the virus quickly, and centers of infection sprang up in widely separated places. Asian flu reached Rhode Island, for example, a month before it was seen in Afghanistan, much closer to its point of origin.

So close was the surveillance that when the disease reached New York City, in August, virologists unhesitatingly identified the first carriers—eight foreign students stepping off a plane. Elsewhere, Asian flu sailed in on destroyers returning from overseas duty.

The value of this medical detective work was borne out when Asian flu eventually subsided. Early detection had given the medical world time to prepare. By October 1, pharmaceutical manufacturers had produced 10 million doses of vaccine, along with extra supplies of antibiotics to ward off the lethal bacterial complications of flu.

The effectiveness of a vaccine depends on how closely the killed virus in the vaccine matches the prevailing wild virus. In tests of perfectly matched vaccines and viruses on volunteer subjects, about 70 per cent of the volunteers are made entirely immune to the flu strain. In actual practice, the effectiveness of flu vaccines varies considerably from year to year. If the wild virus matches the laboratory strain, protection approaches 70 per cent, but if the wild strain drifts, effectiveness drops dramatically.

A killed vaccine is usually administered as an annual injection. Each year people who have had previous contact with the prevailing virus strain, either from a previous year's flu shot or from an infection caused by a similar virus, receive a single dose of vaccine—in effect, a booster for their existing store of antibodies. Those too young to have met the virus previously—the age cutoff varies according to the history of the dominant flu strain—must get two shots about a month apart to build a sufficient reservoir of antibodies.

As both Type A and Type B flu viruses are considered a threat, most influenza vaccines are bivalent, meaning that they protect against two strains. When two variants of Type A are circulating simultaneously, a vaccine may be prepared in a trivalent form, composed of two Type A and one Type B killed viruses. Immunity begins about two weeks after injection, when the antibody level has risen sufficiently to defeat a chance encounter with flu viruses. It generally lasts at close to maximum effectiveness for about six months, but protection lessens sharply thereafter. Since the influenza season generally coincides with the coldest months of the year, most people living in temperate climates get their flu shots in autumn.

Because the immunity conferred by killed-virus vaccines is short-lived and somewhat problematical, virologists continue to search for a better type of vaccine. The most promising research is focused on attenuated, or "live," virus vaccines, which are made with viruses that are specially bred to cause a harmless infection yet trigger flu antibodies. In the past, when such vaccines were used in Japan, China, the Soviet Union and Yugoslavia, the laboratory strains had a dangerous tendency to revert to wild viruses that caused the disease itself. But United States scientists now are experimenting with genetically stable, temperature-sensitive viruses that will grow in the relatively cool temperatures of the nose, but are unable to survive the warmer temperatures in the lungs themselves.

At least in theory, such a live-virus vaccine has several advantages over killed-virus vaccines. It is administered by nose drops or a nasal spray, a route that may stimulate better antibody response in the respiratory secretions, the primary line of defense against influenza. And since live-virus vaccine mimics a natural flu infection, it may give better protection against drifted strains and provide longer immunity than the current killed-virus vaccines.

## Should you get a shot?

Your local public health office or your personal physician can advise you on whether you should get a shot and the proper timing of flu vaccination. The primary candidates for vaccination are individuals who run a high risk of complications: all people over 65, younger people with chronic lung diseases such as asthma, emphysema, chronic bronchitis, tuberculosis and cystic fibrosis, and people suffering from heart disease, kidney disease, diabetes or severe anemia. Cancer and drugs that affect the body's immune system also increase the risk of flu complications and indicate a need for vaccination.

Some otherwise healthy groups are also urged to get vaccinated each fall: people working in the health care field, both because they tend to be exposed to infection more often and because they are so needed in a time of epidemic; providers of essential public services, such as policemen and fire fighters; and military personnel, because they live and work in closed communities where infections spread easily. Pregnant women should discuss the question of vaccination with a physician, and consider the minor risks of a flu shot against the benefits.

On the other hand two possible counterarguments should be considered before you take a shot, even if you fit into one or more of the high-risk categories. If you are allergic to chicken eggs, the medium in which flu vaccines are grown, you should not be vaccinated except under close medical supervision. And if you have an acute infection of any sort or think you may be coming down with one, or have been inoculated for something else in recent weeks, be sure to mention it to the doctor before receiving your shot. You may be advised to postpone your appointment for a few days.

Most people have little or no reaction to the injection. Some—perhaps one in 10—will have slight tenderness, swelling or redness around the puncture; one person in 100 may react for a day or two with a low fever or headache. Popular belief to the contrary, these are not manifestations of mild flu infection, at least in a technical sense. The flu virus in the vaccine is dead, and it cannot infect body cells. However, the body may react to the dead virus particles in much the same way it does to live, infectious ones and cause similar symptoms. Although the result is not flu, it may feel like it.

The most severe reaction to vaccination is Guillain-Barré syndrome, a progressive weakening of muscle strength culminating in paralysis that may last for weeks. This rare disease, which is associated with naturally contracted influenza as well, was connected with flu shots only during the 1976 swine-flu vaccination program in the United States. It has not been seen before or since, but physicians still routinely warn their patients of the remote risk, to avoid legal liability. Guillain-Barré syndrome struck about one in every 100,000 people who were vaccinated during the 1976 program; most of them eventually recovered completely.

Though risk is part of any vaccination program, the dangers of influenza immunization are extremely low—about .001 per cent suffer serious reactions. Measured against the other risks run by high-risk individuals who choose not to have the vaccination and then come down with flu, vaccination wins hands down. But if you experience other than mild symptoms after an inoculation—high fever or continued soreness, for example—consult a physician.

## Putting the vaccines together

Influenza vaccines themselves are a remarkable product of cooperation among physicians, governmental agencies and pharmaceutical companies. Manufacturing them in com-

## Split virus vaccine: a second chance

Although modern influenza vaccines are very effective in preventing the disease, many people remain wary of the shots because they fear the flu-like effects of an inoculation. One attempt to reduce the risk of such effects was the development in the 1960s of a so-called split-virus vaccine, which differed from the standard whole-virus vaccine in its lack of some elements causing reactions. Whole-virus vaccine had been made from the entire virus particle, including both the infinitesimal surface spikes that stimulate immunity and the genetic core, which in an infection causes destruction of body cells. The split-virus type consists almost entirely of the spikes alone, and caused fewer side effects.

Since 1976, the distinction between the two vaccines has been largely academic, at least for adults. New methods of evaluating whole-virus vaccines enabled drug manufacturers to reduce the risk of side effects without sacrificing protective action. However, children are particularly susceptible to side effects. The split-virus type's slightly lower tendency to produce reactions makes it the vaccine of choice for those younger than 13. And many an adult who has resisted getting a flu shot because of an earlier uncomfortable experience is sometimes persuaded to try again with a split-virus vaccine.

Actually both types of vaccine are equal in side effects for most adults. Both are readily available, and most doctors use one or the other routinely. If you have a preference, you will probably have to advise your physician in advance.

*An elderly Californian, Temple Sharkey, winces at the stab of a swine-flu shot during the nationwide vaccination drive of 1976. Planners of the drive made special efforts to vaccinate the elderly, because that segment of the population is particularly vulnerable to fatal complications of flu (page 111).*

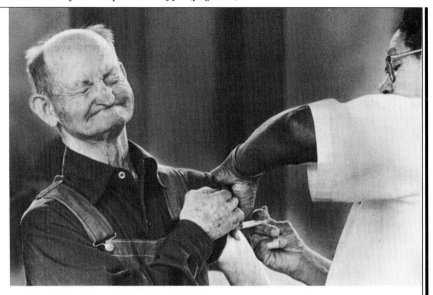

## The epidemic that didn't happen

In January 1976, swine flu—a type of influenza that had not afflicted humans for almost 50 years—broke out at Fort Dix, New Jersey. Several soldiers sickened and one died—and those casualties sparked an unprecedented campaign to immunize every person in the United States. Later that year, the huge program was called off. The epidemic had fizzled, and the vaccine was causing problems.

It was swine flu's dark history that alarmed federal health officials—the 1918-1919 pandemic had started with a strain of swine flu. Scientists warned President Gerald Ford that a new pandemic was possible. In March, Ford declared: "We cannot afford to take a chance with the health of our nation." Congress set aside $135 million to test and buy vaccine.

Soon after the program began, two surprises emerged. Inexplicably, swine flu did not spread. But about 500 of the 46 million who were vaccinated suffered an ugly side effect—a rarely seen paralysis—and 27 of them died. The immunization program was abruptly suspended in December.

The casualties set off a wave of charges that the government had acted rashly in ordering the mass vaccinations. Yet no one had been sure, through the long months of producing and distributing the vaccine, that the swine flu would not become a catastrophic epidemic.

In 1978 a federal study of the mass vaccination was undertaken by impartial medical investigators. They concluded: "We do not yet know enough to predict which new strains will take hold and which won't." If the swine flu had taken hold, many millions of people would have been protected by the vaccine; the deaths of 27 would not have seemed too high a price. Many epidemiologists now agree that the decision to launch the program was the only one possible.

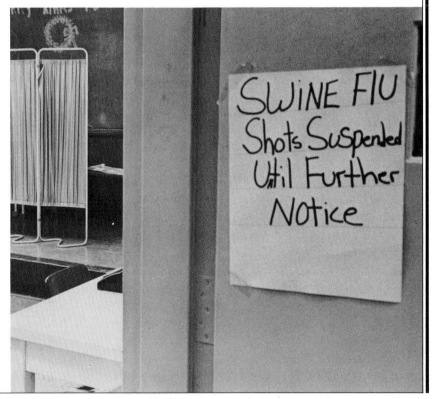

*A sign at a New York City health clinic announces the fate of the swine-flu vaccination plans. Only about 20 per cent of the country's population had been given the vaccine before the program was terminated by federal health officials.*

mercial quantities is like manufacturing automobiles—new models come out every year. The reason for this constant updating, of course, is the continual drift and shift of influenza virus types, and the consequent need to match new vaccines to dominant flu viruses.

To provide manufacturers with the very latest information on flu variants, an international network of nearly 100 surveillance stations, organized under the United Nations' World Health Organization, provides periodic reports on virus types circulating in each station's area. Reports are funneled into centers in London and Atlanta, and these two facilities prepare samples of the dominant influenza strains for each coming influenza season. The samples are distributed to national health services throughout the world; in the United States, for example, the Surgeon General, advised by a panel of flu experts, decides which flu subtypes will be used in commercial vaccines.

In 1953, to standardize identification of flu, the World Health Organization adopted an international system for naming strains and variants. The first recognized influenza strain, the one that prevailed from 1918 to 1957, is tagged H1N1 (for hemagglutinin antigenic type number 1 paired with neuraminidase antigenic type number 1); its variants are specified by the first city or country in which each was found, together with the date of discovery. Thus, A/England/1/51 (H1N1) and A/Denver/1/57 (H1N1) are to some extent related variants of the first strain identified under the system. But the A/Singapore/1/57 (H2N2), which also surfaced in 1957, was a different strain. As it happened, H2N2 was a strain that epidemiologists around the world immediately suspected as a potential troublemaker. They were right: Asian flu, as it came to be known, broke out in China and rapidly swept through Japan, South America, Europe, Africa and the United States.

The mortality rate of Asian flu never approached that of the 1918 flu, perhaps because vaccines reduced the number of susceptible people. The process of getting the vaccines ready is deliberately a last-minute affair, or as much as all concerned dare to make it: The longer the decision makers can wait to assess the influenza scene, the more pre-

cisely the selected vaccine will match the actual virus.

Yet vaccine production remains a tricky business, requiring a long sequence of steps that can be hurried only so much. In the United States, for example, the final decisions that determine the autumn vaccine formula are usually made around the first of March. For these complex decisions, the vaccine panel draws not only upon the past year's data, but also on fragmentary, raw reports of the flu season that is just beginning in the Southern Hemisphere, submitted by stations in such far-flung places as Melbourne, Rio de Janeiro, Montevideo and Johannesburg.

By late spring, samples of concentrated vaccine are ready. If the vaccine meets standards for safety and effectiveness, the government grants the manufacturer approval to go into mass production and distribution.

Substantial quantities of the government-approved vaccines generally become available in September. In years when nothing more than the usual antigenic drift has taken place, the process is fairly orderly. But in those occasional years when a major shift is anticipated—the 1976 scare over the strain called swine flu is a notable example—the "war-mobilization" effort involved can overwhelm all parts of the system. In 1976 the scare proved unwarranted: The shifted virus that epidemiologists thought was coming turned out to be an abortive strain, which died out before it had a chance to do any serious damage.

Preparation for the pandemic that never arrived was not entirely wasted effort. In the United States it excited public concern over the long-term problems of influenza, and it generated a number of changes in the vaccination program. Flu immunization for high-risk groups is now a recognized vaccination program, assuming its place alongside immunization efforts against polio, measles, diphtheria, German measles and other diseases.

The great swine-flu scare also prompted a harder look at reporting and testing systems to see if the time between start-up and delivery of licensed vaccines could be shortened. And finally, it promoted research into alternatives and reinforcements to vaccines, promising better protection against this disease in the future. ✻

# In World War I: defeat by disease

When, in late August, the second, deadly wave of the 1918 influenza pandemic swept across the United States, soldiers training at Camp Devens, Massachusetts, were among the first to fall. By the time Dr. William Henry Welch, the nation's preeminent pathologist, reached the scene on September 23, the 45,000-man camp was a shambles: A continuous line of men was reporting sick, and 12,000 had been hospitalized, 1,900 of them with pneumonia. On the day Colonel Welch arrived, 63 men died; soon the toll had climbed to 90 a day.

In the camp morgue Colonel Welch opened up the chest of a dead soldier. The cause of death was obvious: The victim's lungs, which should have been as light as a child's balloon, looked like heavy sacks filled with a thin, bloody, frothy fluid. Welch, a pathologist hardened by a half century of autopsies, had never seen that pattern of disease. "This must be some new kind of infection," he said, "or plague."

Within weeks the pandemic raced through the country and across the Atlantic to Europe, killing civilians and soldiers alike. In New York City 19,000 died, and in a single New York borough 2,000 bodies lay unburied. Doctors making house calls were mobbed by terrified flu victims, and ambulance drivers found patients alone in their homes, abandoned by relatives who feared contagion.

But the military bore the brunt of the disease. As infectious flu carriers intermixed with fresh contingents of healthy recruits, the contagion spread. The Army fought as best it could. On some bases, water fountains were sterilized hourly with blowtorches, quarantines were enforced at gunpoint, and recruits marched 20 feet apart. But such precautions, devised in ignorance of the nature of the flu virus, did little good. Before the pandemic ended, influenza struck 734,000 soldiers and killed 23,559—one third of the total U.S. casualties during the War.

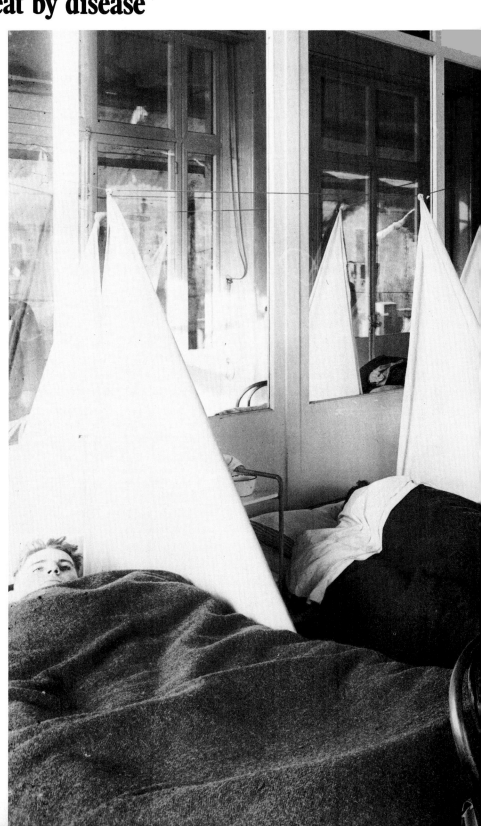

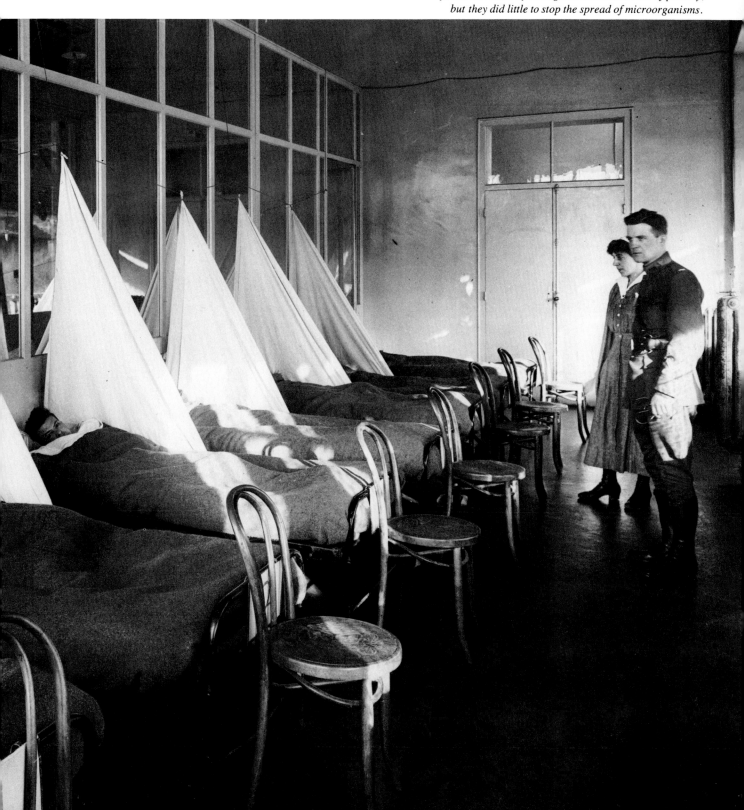

*Two months after the Armistice, rows of flu-stricken soldiers fill a military hospital at Aix-les-Bains in southeast France, while a U.S. Army doctor and nurse stand by to ease the symptoms of a disease they could not prevent or cure. Temporary partitions and fabric screens may have given the men a sense of privacy, but they did little to stop the spread of microorganisms.*

# Emergency care for the first casualties

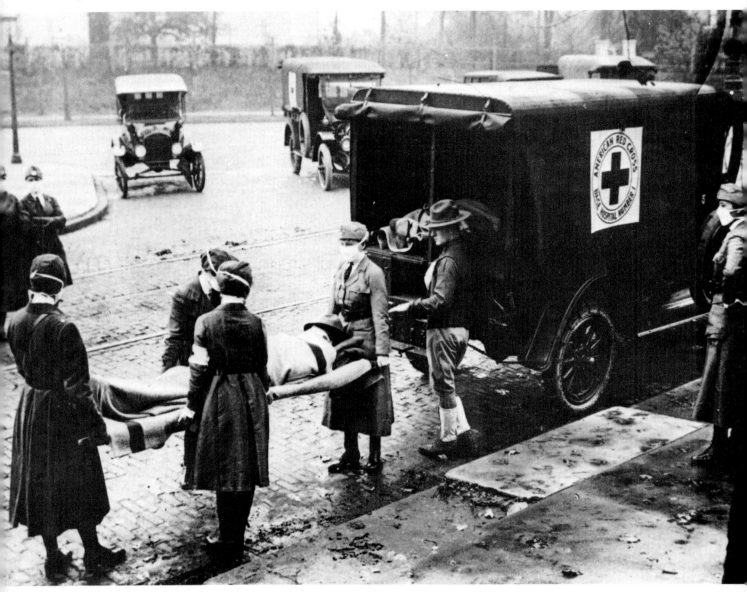

*Red Cross workers like the ones in this ambulance unit in St. Louis, Missouri, offered nursing and administrative and moral support at overburdened military hospitals. Many civilian volunteers died of flu or of exhaustion brought on by overwork.*

*A doctor and nurse at Fort Porter, near Buffalo, New York, check one hollow-eyed patient's progress. Hoping to reduce contagion in this crowded facility, hospital authorities instituted the practice of arranging the beds so that each victim's feet were next to his neighbor's head.*

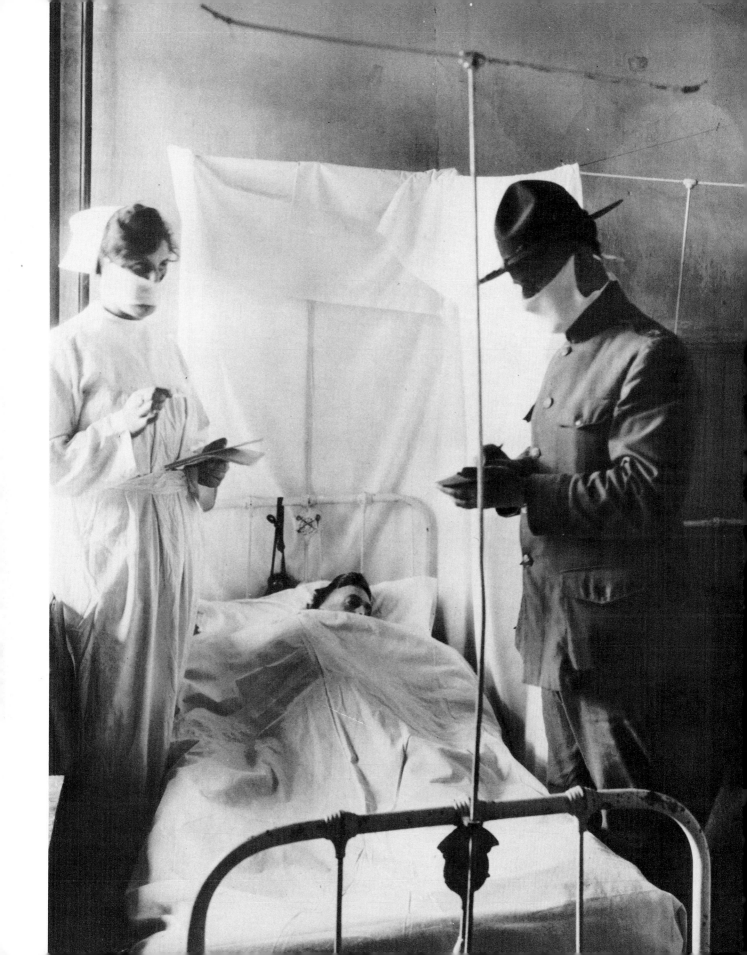

# A futile struggle to limit contagion

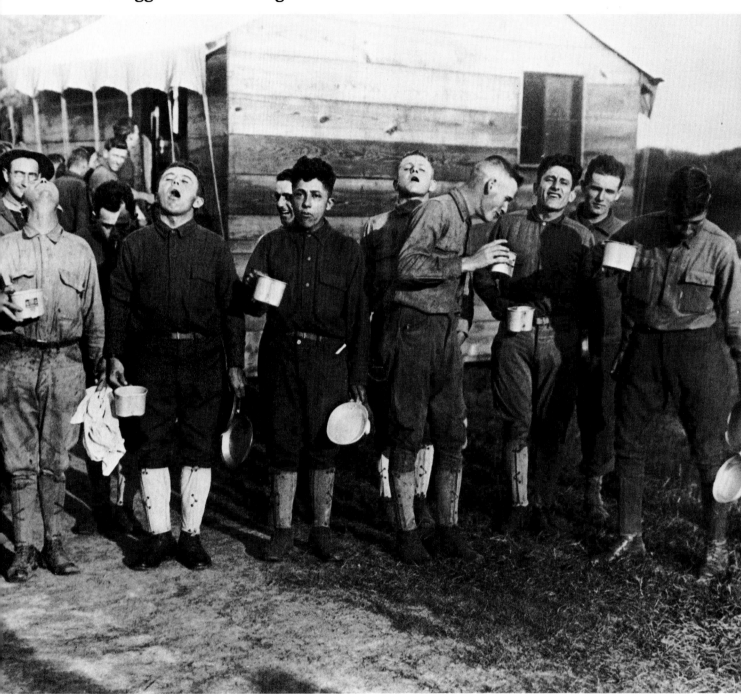

*At New Jersey's Camp Dix, recruits with mess cups in hand
go through a mandatory ritual of gargling with salt water before
falling in for a meal at the mess hall (rear). Nonetheless,
admissions at the Dix base hospital soared to 2,358 within the first
month of the pandemic, and 183 men died.*

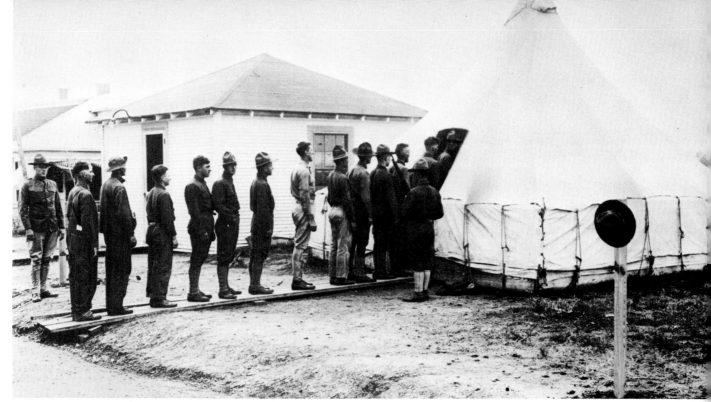

*Air servicemen at Love Field, Dallas, Texas (above), wait patiently outside the medic's tent for a daily throat spray. At left, a medical corpsman sprays each patient from a common atomizer. At best, this attempt at disease control had no effect at all. At worst, it may have spread the virus.*

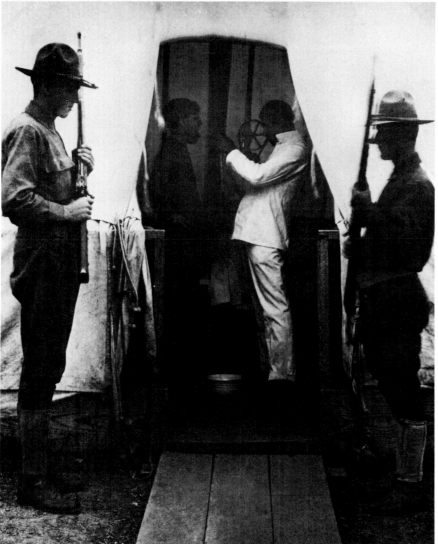

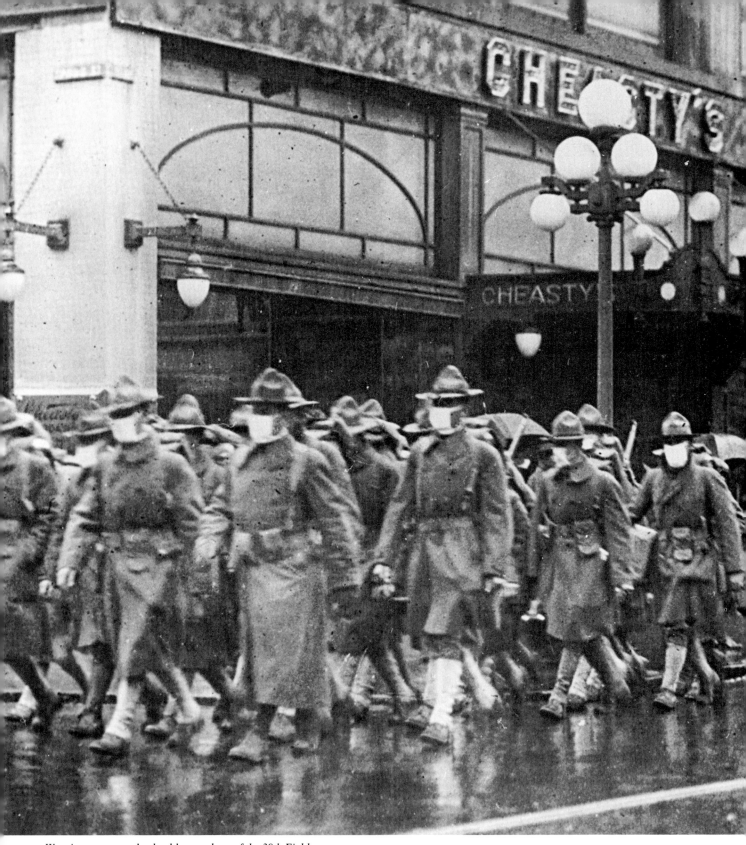

*Wearing gauze masks, healthy members of the 39th Field
Artillery Regiment, stationed at Camp Lewis, Washington, march
smartly through the deserted streets of Seattle in the winter of
1918. They and their officers may have felt they were taking no
chances with flu viruses on that cold, wet day, but U.S.
health officers have since declared the masks almost useless.*

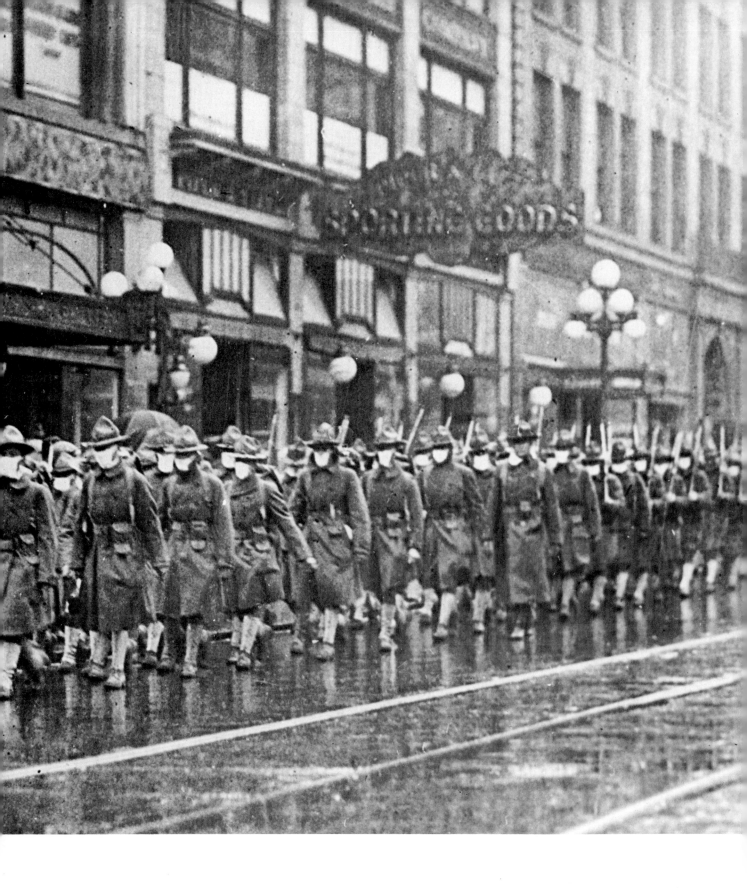

# Last-ditch battles against an implacable foe

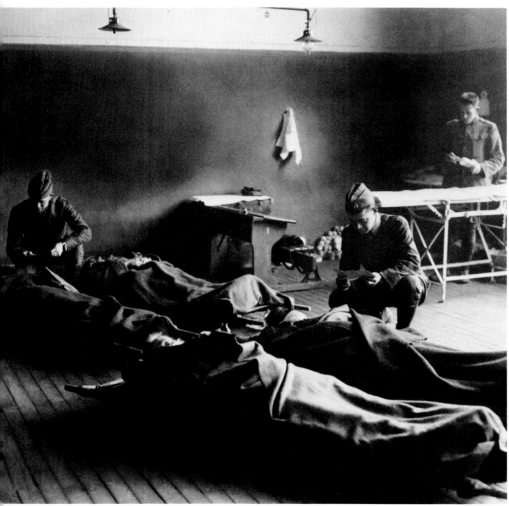

*Doctors review the records of four new stretcher admissions
in a schoolroom in Hollerich, Luxembourg — a makeshift hospital
typical of the best the Army could provide in some war zones.*

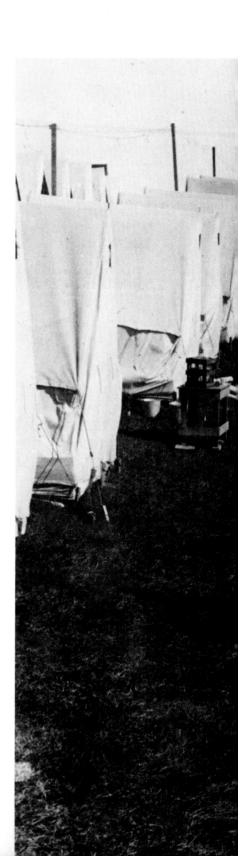

*At an emergency unit set up by the U.S. military in Brookline,
Massachusetts — a tent city on the grounds of a civilian
hospital — nurses attend their patients outdoors. In September
1918 this 1,600-bed sick bay was served by an informal
water-supply system that tapped into town fire hydrants. By mid-
October the case load had fallen sufficiently to move the
remaining patients to more substantial base hospitals elsewhere.*

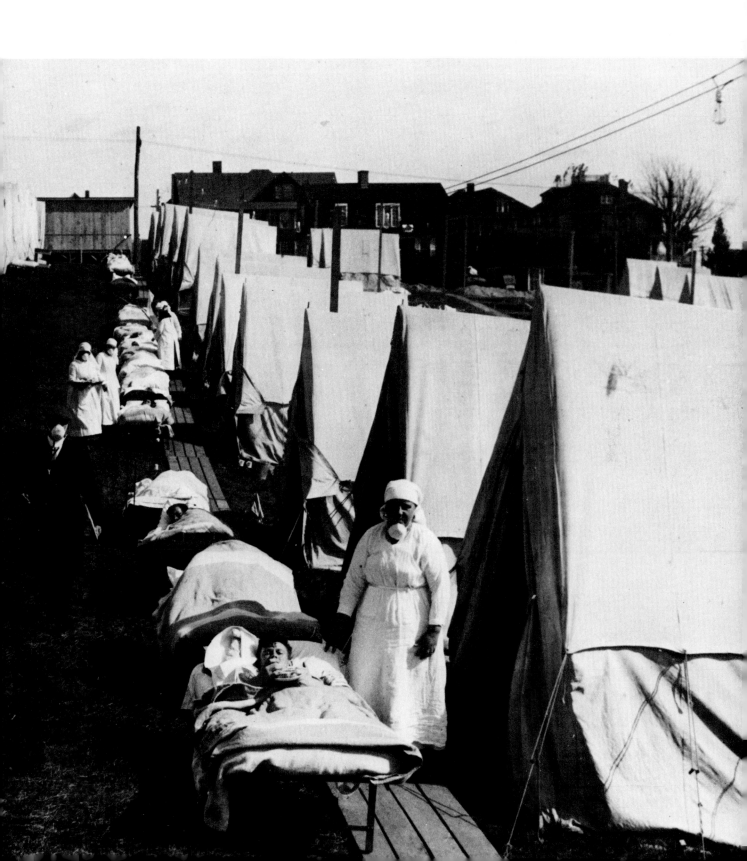

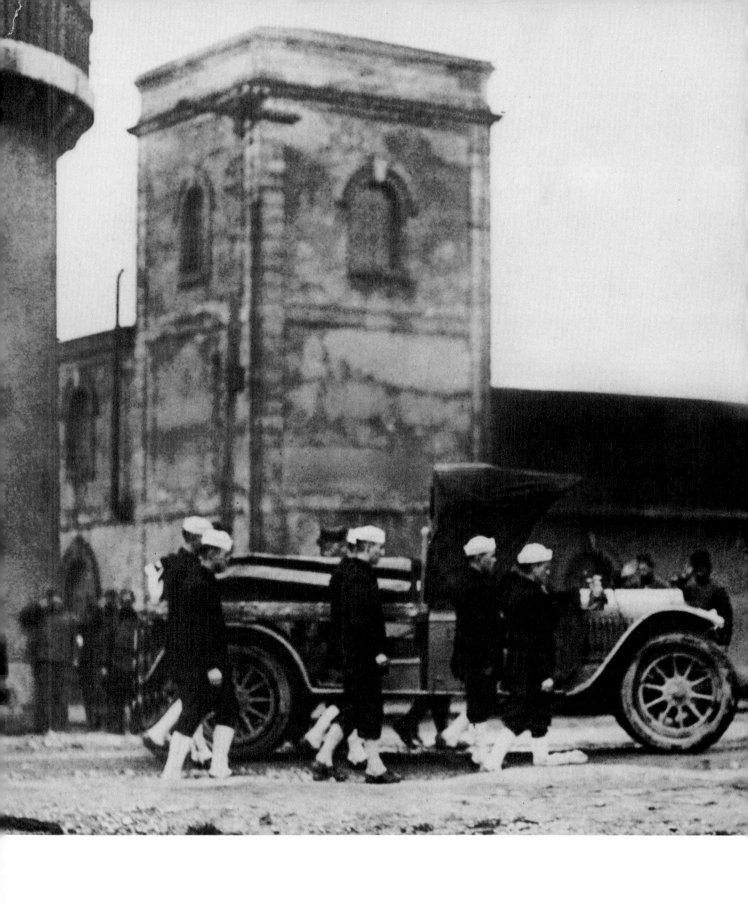

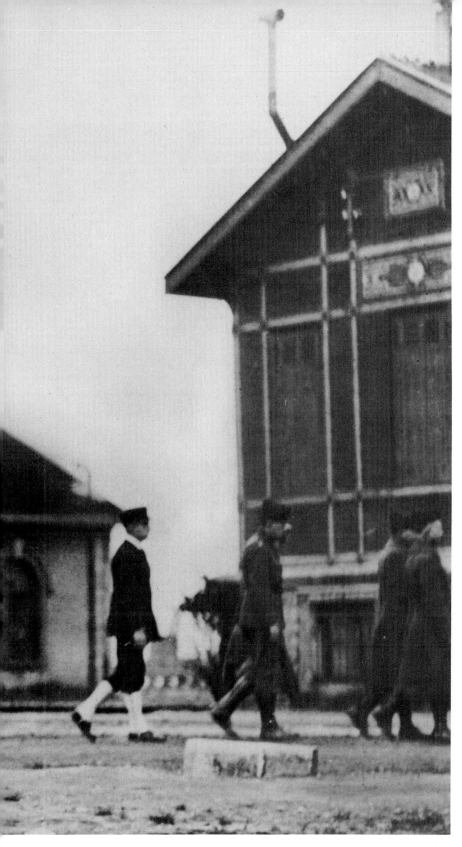

In February 1919, three months after the signing of the Armistice, an honor guard escorts the bodies of two countrymen to burial at a port near Bordeaux, where doughboys were massed for embarkation to the United States. "Every soldier who has died from influenza," said General Peyton March, the Army Chief of Staff, "has just as surely played his part as his comrade who died on the battlefield."

# CHAPTER 5

# The tantalizing quest for a cure

**Controversial prescription from a Nobel Prize chemist**
**Does vitamin C really work?**
**A man-made substance that could prevent colds**
**New drugs that make viruses go away**

In the first flush of excitement following the discovery of cold viruses in the 1950s, it seemed only a matter of time until a vaccine would render the cold at least as avoidable as influenza. Unfortunately, no such vaccine has been developed, and no one with inside information holds much hope that it will be in the near future. But there are, just over the horizon, subtler ways of combating this ancient human enemy than the head-on attack of an all-purpose vaccine.

The difficulties of devising a cold vaccine stem from the complexities of assembling a brew that could protect against all or even most of the 200 or so known cold viruses. If a vaccine to counter existing viruses was developed, widespread immunity to them could lead to the emergence of hundreds of other, perhaps more potent, types. Such genetic changes are already thought to be a factor in the alterations that occur in influenza-A viruses, and similar changes may have been behind the sequence of events noticed in the early 1970s when the armed forces started using a cold vaccine to prevent outbreaks on military bases *(page 52)*. The vaccine was compounded to combat the viruses most prevalent at these installations and it was successful. But two other types of viruses have since begun infecting small numbers of recruits, and scientists are concerned about the possibility that serious outbreaks of respiratory infection could return.

While the promise of a cold vaccine has faded, the potential for infection has been increasing. As the world becomes more populous and people live and work in ever-closer proximity, breathing the same air, touching surfaces that hundreds, perhaps thousands, of others have touched the same day, the opportunity for transmission of respiratory infections continues to grow. However, there are alternatives to a future of colds and more colds, of succeeding generations spending their days clutching damp handkerchiefs. The new solutions to old problems are coming from new knowledge, acquired only in recent decades, of virus activity.

Once the secrets of the basic chemicals of living cells began to be deciphered in the years following World War II, the mysteries of the body's immunological processes could be revealed and the life cycles of specific viruses plotted. Then it became possible to see how those life cycles might be interfered with and their ill effects blocked. Various natural and synthetic substances have now been found that promise antiviral power, although their value is not yet fully established. It is no longer unrealistic to expect that antiviral medicines able to prevent or stop colds and flu may someday be available at the corner drugstore.

Among the cold and flu fighters now being studied and clinically tested, three have aroused the most interest. One is a synthetic that inhibits the reproduction of certain influenza viruses. Another is a natural component of the immune system, the all-purpose virus stopper interferon. The third is the common and essential ingredient in fresh fruits and vegetables, vitamin C.

The notion that vitamin C might be helpful in fighting the common cold and flu has been dallied with since shortly after the vitamin was isolated, in 1928, by Albert Szent-Györgyi,

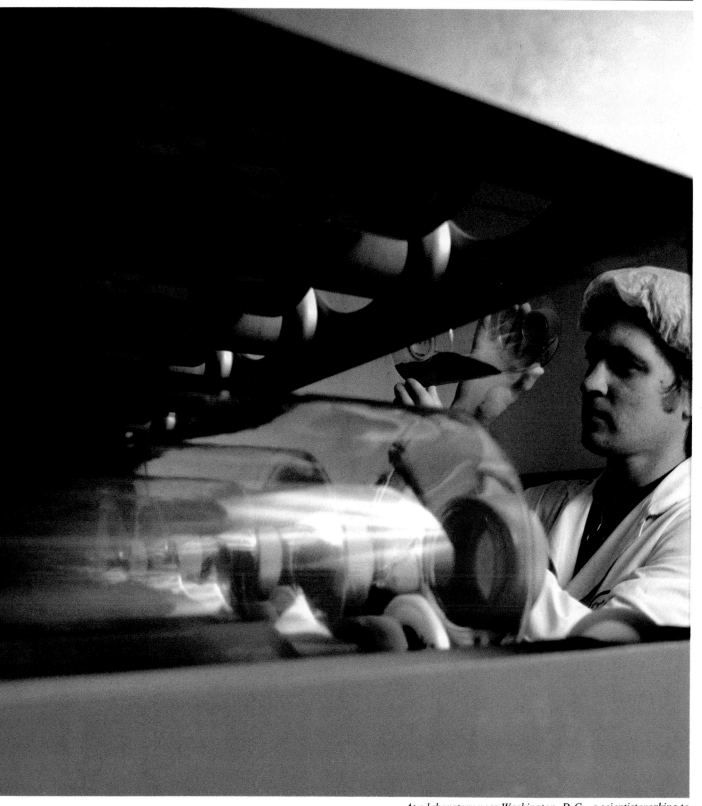

*At a laboratory near Washington, D.C., a scientist working to produce the virus-fighting protein interferon examines human skin cells growing in red brews of nutrients. The cells make interferon by an incredibly slow and costly process —60 million of these bottles yield about an ounce of the substance.*

138

the Hungarian-born biochemist who later won the Nobel Prize for Physiology and Medicine. Almost half a century later, however, the pros and cons of taking vitamin C in huge amounts—150 times more than is generally considered necessary in food—became a matter of lively controversy.

## Controversial prescription from a Nobel Prize chemist

In 1970 a book entitled *Vitamin C and the Common Cold* was published. It made a stir because of the eminence of its author, Linus Pauling, the brilliant Stanford University chemist who has a penchant for antiestablishment causes. Pauling has won two Nobel Prizes: one in 1954 for his discoveries of the natural laws governing the structure of complex chemical compounds, and one in 1962 for his antiwar activities.

Pauling is not a physician. He did not conduct any experiments of his own, but used the results of several tests done by others, some as long ago as 1939. He then derived his recommendations for preventing colds from chemical principles and personal experience. In his best-selling book and in subsequent writings, he asserted that people who supplement their normal diet with very large doses of vitamin C—1,000 to 2,000 milligrams, about $1/14$ ounce—every day, and take additional massive doses of 4,000 to 10,000 milligrams when they have a cold will suffer fewer, shorter and milder colds. He predicted an average 45 per cent reduction in the incidence of colds and a 60 per cent reduction in days of illness for those who followed his regimen.

Vitamin C, Pauling pointed out, was known to be essential in promoting a chain of chemical reactions leading to the formation of collagen, the threadlike material that cements tissue cells together. "Part of the effectiveness of vitamin C against the common cold, influenza and other viral diseases," he postulated, "can be attributed to its action in strengthening the intercellular cement and in this way preventing or hindering the motion of the virus particles through the tissue and into the cells." Pauling also suspected that vitamin C was involved in the synthesis and activity of that natural virus-fighting agent, interferon.

Pauling based his argument for large doses of vitamin C on the fact that human beings, unlike most animals, cannot produce vitamin C in their bodies and must get all of it from food. This shortcoming, he believed, was caused by an evolutionary mistake that reduced resistance to infection.

Sometime in early human history, said Pauling, Homo sapiens or his immediate antecedent underwent some sort of genetic change that ended his ability to synthesize the vitamin. So long as humans lived in tropical or subtropical climates, where they naturally ate large amounts of raw vegetables and fruits rich in vitamin C, the lost ability was not missed. But few if any people eat in this fashion any more, even in summer months, when such foods are readily available. And in winter the majority of people are almost entirely dependent for their vitamin C on cooked and preserved foods, which may lose much of their vitamin content during preparation. It is no coincidence, Pauling declared, that the season of greatest respiratory infection is also the season of least intake of vitamin C from food.

This reasoning led Pauling to a startling prediction of an idyllic, cold-free world: If large segments of the population raised their vitamin C consumption to the levels he recommended, and if people would isolate themselves when suffering from colds, cold viruses might in time be driven from civilized company and cold infections would disappear altogether for lack of a cooperative host.

The treatment Pauling prescribed became a cause célèbre. In the years following publication of his book, the consumption of vitamin C tablets and liquid concentrates in the United States skyrocketed.

The medical community remained skeptical if not downright hostile. Most researchers rejected Pauling's recommendations as scientifically unsound—the experiments he drew on, critics said, were flawed. They also warned that too little was known about the possible toxic effects of massive doses of vitamin C to risk casual self-medication of the sort Pauling recommended. Not surprisingly, popular feeling grew that the critics were being cynical or reactionary, their warnings tinged perhaps with professional jealousy because the long-awaited cold cure had come not from someone in the medical establishment but from an outsider. Pauling appeared to be a David challenging an army of Goliaths.

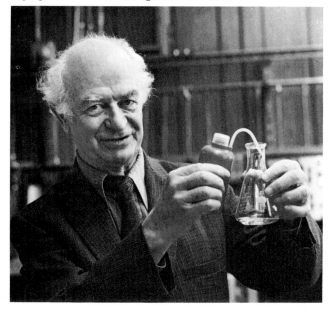

*Nobel Prize-winning chemist Linus Pauling, an advocate of vitamin C as a cold preventive, tests a urine sample for traces of the vitamin, in his laboratory at Menlo Park, California. Pauling believes that massive doses of vitamin C reinforce collagen, the connective substance surrounding human cells, thus helping it to shield the cells against cold viruses.*

In the years since the controversy first arose, researchers have studied vitamin C as both a preventive drug and a therapeutic drug for colds, using more sophisticated research techniques, larger population samples and newer knowledge of the immune system and of viruses than were available before. Though all the evidence is not yet in and important questions remain unanswered, it is now clear that the truth of vitamin C's effect on colds lies somewhere between the extremes of panacea and total irrelevance. There is some evidence that large doses of vitamin C can help ameliorate colds. The key question is how much they help. The disease is a minor one, and the treatment must be worth its costs in effort and risks. Before anyone consumes a substance to prevent or cure an illness as mild as the common cold, he should be certain it will indeed do him good—and no harm.

## A vitamin C primer

A great deal has been learned about vitamin C in the centuries since physicians first realized that fresh fruits and vegetables were somehow vital to human health. It is, first of all, a white crystalline chemical, a simple compound named ascorbic acid—having the same form whether its origins are natural or synthetic. Vitamin C is absorbed into the system through the small intestine and is soluble in water, so that it can enter body fluids easily. Very little of it is stored in humans; consequently it must be replenished by steady intake, preferably every day. Quantities in excess of current needs are eliminated rapidly in the urine.

The primary—and most obvious—need for vitamin C is for help in maintaining the continuing process of growth and bodily repair. A lack of sufficient vitamin C causes scurvy, a debilitating failure of the growth and repair process marked by weakness, anemia, bleeding gums, loss of teeth and, ultimately, death.

Scurvy, a disease seen only in unusual circumstances today, was a major killer from prehistoric times into the 19th Century. First noted by Hippocrates in ancient Greece, the disease is one of the few caused solely by lack of a single nutrient. Long associated with social upheavals that disrupted supplies of fresh fruits and vegetables, scurvy wiped out vast numbers of people during wars and sieges. Its depredations were recorded by physicians and chroniclers during the Crusades, and in medieval times it was a recurring visitor to Northern Europe during the long winter months.

During the great Age of Exploration, which began in the late 15th Century, when ships started to make journeys lasting many months between stops for supplies, scurvy became an occupational hazard for sailors. As early as 1535, the French explorer Jacques Cartier and his men were introduced to a cure for scurvy. Virtually the entire crew, near death from the disease, was saved by Iroquois Indians in Newfoundland who fed them a brew made from the bark and leaves of local trees. Dutch and English sailors of the 16th Century also learned how to prevent and cure scurvy by eating fruits and juices.

British Admiral Sir Richard Hawkins wrote in 1593 of 10,000 deaths from scurvy that he knew of personally, and stated, ''That which I have seen most fruitful for this sickness is sower oranges and lemons.'' Yet for two more centuries scurvy killed additional tens of thousands of sailors, and European medicine seemed helpless to do anything about it.

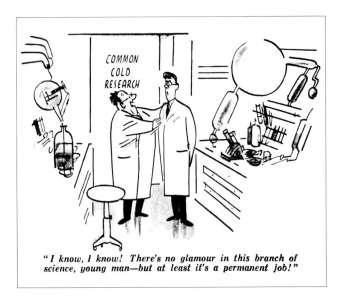

*"I know, I know! There's no glamour in this branch of science, young man—but at least it's a permanent job!"*

Finally, in 1747, a British Navy doctor, James Lind, conducted well-controlled therapeutic tests that demonstrated the specific ability of oranges and lemons to cure scurvy. He published a conclusive report of his findings in 1753, recommending daily rations of lemon or orange juice for all crew members on long voyages. Unfortunately, the British Admiralty was unimpressed with his discovery and did nothing.

The value of Lind's findings was dramatically demonstrated by the experience of the brilliant seafarer Captain James Cook, who, beginning in 1768, made three explorations of the Pacific Ocean without losing a single crew member to scurvy. Cook adhered to Lind's principles, ordering a daily portion for all hands of "sour krout"—or fresh fruits and vegetables, from supplies renewed whenever the crew went ashore. Although Cook is remembered today for his achievements as a navigator and explorer, during his own lifetime he won greatest fame and was made a Fellow of the Royal Society because of his contributions to health.

Nevertheless, it took 41 years from the time of Dr. Lind's report, and perhaps 10,000 more agonizing deaths of British sailors, before the Admiralty saw fit, in 1794, to issue a supply of lemon juice to a squadron leaving on a 23-week cruise. And though this timid first step of the bureaucracy was a complete success, it took another 10 years for British officialdom to enforce daily portions of lemon juice for all Naval crews. Only then did scurvy disappear from the ranks of the British Navy. Incredibly, the British Board of Trade did not apply the same regulations to merchant ships until another 50 years had passed.

Although the fruit juice recommended by Navy physicians came from lemons, the sailors became known as limeys because—possibly to boost consumption of limes from Britain's West Indian colonies—lime juice was substituted early in the 19th Century as the standard antiscurvy ration. Scurvy reappeared in the British Navy on 19th Century expeditions to the North Pole. Not until after the active antiscurvy agent, vitamin C, was identified in 1928 did it become clear that limes were only half as effective against scurvy as lemons.

A mere 10 milligrams of vitamin C in the daily diet is enough to keep scurvy at bay. How much additional is needed for other bodily functions is not yet precisely known, although nutritionists have over the years examined vitamin C's behavior in the body to find the answers. By giving volunteers doses of the vitamin that have been made harmlessly radioactive, they can trace the radioactivity and follow vitamin C as it moves through the body, thereby establishing the patterns of bodily processing, storage, uptake by the blood, and elimination. These patterns become the basis for establishing healthful vitamin C levels in an overall set of dietary standards, the recommended dietary allowances promulgated by government health authorities. In the United States these standards are based on measurements of the daily quantity sufficient to prevent scurvy, to replenish amounts chemically processed by the body in 24 hours, and to maintain an adequate reserve against the unlikely circumstance of an extended lapse in normal vitamin C intake.

The recommendations vary slightly from country to country, primarily because different countries use slightly different criteria for measurement. In West Germany, for example, the daily recommendation for adults is 75 milligrams in "food as purchased." The United Kingdom stipulates a minimum—30 milligrams per day for adults. In Denmark, Finland, East Germany, Japan and Czechoslovakia, the recommendations for adults are 45, 30, 70, 50 and 50 milligrams per day, respectively.

In the United States the suggested amount, called a recommended dietary allowance, or RDA, for healthy teenagers and adults is 60 milligrams, for young children 45 milligrams, for infants 35 milligrams. Pregnant women, particularly those in the second and third trimesters, need an extra 20 milligrams a day. Nursing mothers need as much as 40 additional milligrams daily, virtually all of which is passed on to the suckling infant. Labels on processed foods generally express vitamin content as a percentage of the RDA contained.

Anyone eating a moderately well-balanced diet will more than meet the RDA for vitamin C. A single eight-ounce glass of fresh, canned or frozen orange juice, for example, provides approximately 120 milligrams of vitamin C, 20 per cent more than the RDA for nursing mothers and twice as much as the average adult needs. In addition to citrus fruits, fresh fruits of many sorts are rich in vitamin C, as are such fresh vegetables as broccoli, Brussels sprouts, turnips, and red and green peppers. (Albert Szent-Györgyi delightedly noted that the vitamin he discovered was richly provided by the distinctive seasoning of his native Hungary: paprika.) Even cooked vegetables and fruits—whether fresh, frozen or canned—will supply significant amounts of vitamin C if they are heated briefly, at moderate temperatures and for immediate consumption. Frozen and canned vegetables and fruits, if picked at peak maturity and properly processed with little delay, may actually retain more vitamin C than fresh counterparts that have been stored poorly or for long periods.

Although health authorities around the world are in general if not perfect agreement on optimum amounts of vitamin C, Linus Pauling has disputed the consensus, contending that the present RDAs are too low to help the body fight colds. The obvious way to find out if he is right is to test his thesis: Give experimental groups large doses of the vitamin and see if they catch fewer colds than other people. This has been done. The results are controversial, as such tests are maddeningly subject to error. The challenge is to design a study so flawless that even the most biased opponent can repeat it with his own staff and subjects and get the same results.

The more that researchers learn about the complexities of colds, the harder it is for them to create such unchallengeable tests. If one group of volunteers gets measured doses of vitamin C and a second, control, group takes doses of a substance known to be innocuous—a placebo—the two groups must be virtually identical in age distribution, male-female ratio, general state of health, past experience of colds, general diet, smoking habits, stress levels, family composition and work environment. As the test proceeds, the dropout rates of the two groups must remain substantially the same. The sample size and the duration of the test must be great enough to rule out chance variations that have nothing to do with the effect of the vitamin or the placebo. For example, if the group includes hundreds of individuals, the impact of one person's cold on the total test results will be far less likely to tilt scores one way or the other than the impact of such an event in a group of just 10 people.

Another essential for a reputable test is a safeguard against psychologically induced error, for medical experimenters and their subjects are very vulnerable to self-deception. Subjects and test administrators alike must be kept completely in the dark about who is and who is not receiving the active drug. This technique, known as a double-blind study, is never more necessary than in investigating colds and flu.

Evaluation of respiratory infections depends on slippery data—the subjective views of the sufferer and the investigator, who must record what are at best inexact and unquantifiable symptoms. For some test subjects, the psychosomatic effect of knowing they are getting vitamin C rather than a placebo will be enough to make them feel better. Similarly, subjects who learn that they have only a placebo to ward off infection may in some way become more susceptible to sickness or at least tend subconsciously to give more importance to the symptoms they do experience. The test administrator, who may well begin his research with an unacknowledged bias for or against the test substance, may subconsciously permit that bias to get in the way of a fair evaluation, too.

In a classic double-blind test a system of coded numbers, known only to a third party, matches volunteers and medications, keeping everyone on an equally infirm footing. Fur-

## A 30-year crusade against the common cold

"To write a book about colds is rather like writing a review of a play in the middle of the first act," noted Sir Christopher Andrewes, Great Britain's "Grand Old Man of Virology"—good-humoredly portrayed in a British cartoon *(right)* as a knight in shining armor attacking the common cold, his mount a ferret used for tests, his weapon a syringe. When Sir Christopher retired after some 30 years' work with cold—and flu—viruses, his book remained to be written, but knowledge about colds that does exist is due largely to his efforts.

In 1946 Sir Christopher organized the Common Cold Unit in Salisbury, England. With human volunteers as well as animals like the ferret in the cartoon, the quest began in earnest. After 14 years of testing countless throat swabs, nose washings, sneeze bags and blood samples, the unit succeeded in growing cold viruses in cultures approximating conditions in the human nose. Eventually the unit was able to confirm that colds were caused not by one virus but by many.

These and other accomplishments allowed subsequent research to focus more sharply on the natural history of colds, the way viruses get from one person to another, the defenses the body has against them, and the duration of immunity—questions that remain only partially answered.

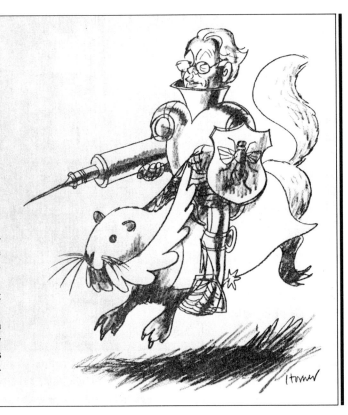

ther, great care is taken to make the placebo and the medication similar in size, color and taste, so that no one involved has any basis for identifying the substance until after the results are tabulated. One experiment with vitamin C ran into problems because of a simple error that was discovered only after the experiment ended: The researchers tested the sharply acid vitamin against a bland-tasting placebo. When they later asked the subjects if they were able to guess which they had been administered, several said they were. (Those subjects were eliminated from the results, which, thus corrected, indicated no special value for the vitamin.)

Finally, a proper test should include a reasonable certainty of compliance on the part of subjects. Many "open" tests depend on unsupervised volunteers, who have to remember to take a prescribed dose two or three times a day, week after

week, and to keep accurate records of their experiences. More reliable on this score are trials administered in a "closed" situation such as a school, a prison or a common place of employment, where supervisory personnel can oversee the administration of substances, the general diet and the reporting of illness. However, a closed environment introduces errors of its own. The special nature of the situation raises doubts about the relevance of participants' reactions to those of the general population.

The complexities of modern drug testing and the potential for misinterpretation that lurks in all tests make it clear that seeing should not always be believing when it comes to judging the efficacy of vitamin C. Persuasive though Aunt Millie's unfailing success with vitamin C or mustard plaster may be, her miracles could derive from any number of circumstances, including hyperactive cilia, a super immune system or a natural bent for looking on the bright side, none of which owe anything to vitamins or the bracing sting of mustard.

**Does vitamin C really work?**

In 1975 Dr. Michael H. M. Dykes, Senior Scientist with the American Medical Association's Department of Drugs, and Paul Meier, Professor in the Departments of Statistics and Pharmacological and Physical Sciences at the University of Chicago, reviewed the eight studies done since 1938 that supported the usefulness of vitamin C in treating the common cold. They found only one experiment that they considered well designed and of some validity—a study done by Dr. Terence Anderson, then Professor of Epidemiology in the Faculty of Medicine, University of Toronto.

In the winter of 1971 and 1972, Dr. Anderson set out to test Pauling's 1,000-milligram-to-4,000-milligram treatment on half of 1,000 volunteers, the other half being given a well-disguised placebo in a 14-week double-blind study. He found that vitamin C was of little or no help in preventing colds or in bringing them to an early halt. But he was surprised to discover data suggesting that the vitamin might have some effect on the severity of colds as measured by the amount of time test subjects stayed home or out of work because of illness. Among subjects who caught cold during the trial, those who used vitamin C were disabled 30 per cent fewer days than those taking the placebo. Such a difference could not have arisen by chance, but its practical effect was minor: Vitamin C users were laid up an average of 1.3 days with their colds, while those in the control group were out for an average 1.9 days.

In a second study conducted the following year, Anderson and his colleagues took a different tack, to determine if vitamin C helped as a preventive or a therapeutic remedy; they also tested higher and lower doses. They found that vitamin C had insignificant effect if used as preventive medication alone or as therapeutic treatment alone. Only the few volunteers administered vitamin C as a preventive who then caught cold and received therapeutic doses had milder symptoms. Even more important, the researchers found that small daily

doses were as effective as larger ones up to 2,000 milligrams.

In a third test a year later, Dr. Anderson cut the vitamin C dosage to 500 milligrams a week plus 1,500 milligrams on the first day of symptoms and 1,000 milligrams on each of the next four days. As in the first two studies, Anderson found no significant difference in cold susceptibility or in the duration of symptoms, but some of the symptoms—fever, chills, bodily aches and pains—were less severe. Little relief was noted in such localized symptoms as inflammation, nasal blockage, sneezing and coughing.

Like Dr. Anderson's three studies, virtually all testing of vitamin C since Linus Pauling published his theories has been based on observations of people and their experience with colds after taking the substance. But a few experiments have been done using laboratory cultures or animals to see whether some explanation might be found for the reduced severity of colds encountered in experiments such as Dr. Anderson's. These experiments, too, indicate that vitamin C might help fight cold viruses.

Working with laboratory cultures at the University of Rochester Medical School, Drs. John P. Manzella and Norbert Roberts Jr. found that adding vitamin C to the cultures had a significant effect on an important component of the immune system—the white cells known as macrophages, or big eaters *(Chapter 2)*, that consume infectious agents. When vitamin C was applied in concentrations equal to those in the blood of volunteers in earlier clinical studies, the big eaters became more active.

Other researchers discovered evidence of an effect on interferon. If mice received vitamin C supplements in their drinking water, they subsequently produced greater amounts of interferon when exposed to viral infection. Test-tube experiments with artificial interferon inducers *(page 148)* also indicated greater interferon production by cells when vitamin C was added to the culture.

These results give some support to Pauling's thesis: Vitamin C helps. Whether it helps enough to warrant its use is another matter. Dr. Anderson and most other researchers in the field have stated that vitamin C's apparent ability to alleviate the severity of some cold symptoms does not justify

# Blocking colds with iodine facial tissues

''Killer hankies''—ordinary facial tissues treated with iodine to kill viruses—may someday help block the spread of colds. The hankies seemed to work when tested by their inventor, Elliot C. Dick of the University of Wisconsin, in experiments at McMurdo Station, the main American scientific base in Antarctica.

Dick chose Antarctica not for its cruel climate—which apparently has little effect on colds—but for its isolation. The 60 scientists and military personnel on long-term duty there rarely suffer from colds because they are completely cut off from virus carriers—until the annual winter fly-in brings in some 150 additional men and women for a five-week stay. The respiratory illnesses that some newcomers carry with them are the only such ailments introduced to the community during each test period—and the rate of infection soars.

The experiments began during the antarctic winter of 1979. Each day everyone at McMurdo received pocket-sized packages of the tissues, with instructions to blow his nose with one, wipe his hands and face with another, then wipe both face and hands with fresh tissues every hour. Four days after the killer hankies went into use, the number of new colds reported daily dropped from an average of 4.3 to 1.7. If subsequent tests produce similar results, Dick foresees the possibility that virus-killing handkerchiefs will be put into use in schools, hospitals and other places where people are confined in close quarters.

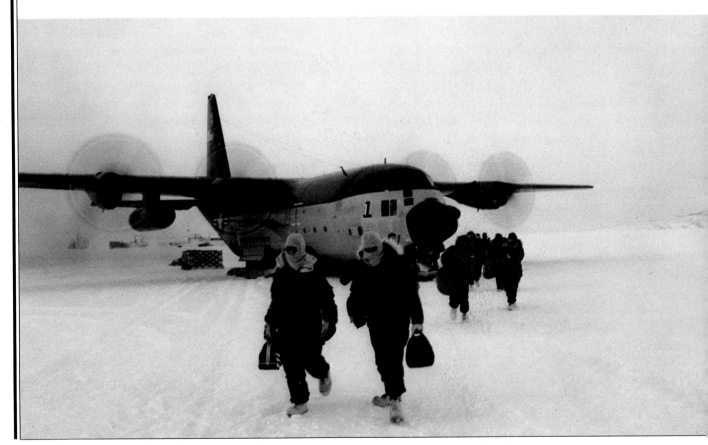

*Military personnel and civilian scientists disembark from a skiplane to begin a five-week tour of duty at McMurdo Station. Their isolation made them ideal subjects for a test of antivirus tissues as a means of blocking the spread of colds.*

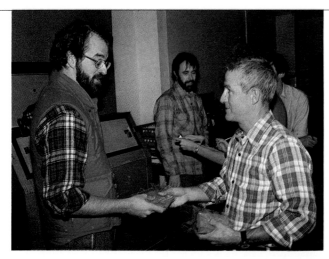

*Elliot C. Dick (right) hands out packages of killer hankies to the chow line at the McMurdo mess hall; as he distributes the hankies, he asks about signs of a cold or other respiratory illness, and an assistant (partly obscured) records the answers. Each participant in Dick's experiment received two packs of 10 tissues each day.*

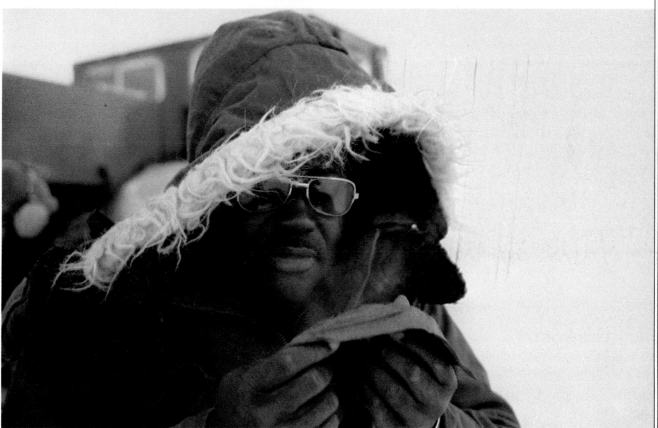

*His breath condensing in the antarctic cold—the air temperature was -20° F.—a soldier in the air-transport crew prepares to use one of the brown-stained antivirus tissues that reduced the spread of colds in trials at the South Pole.*

taking large doses of it for colds day after day, year after year, particularly when many questions remain as to its potential for harm.

Although most people seem able to tolerate large doses of vitamin C and eliminate excess amounts from their bodies routinely, some serious side effects are at least theoretically possible among the minority who cannot regularly clear large amounts of the vitamin from their systems. When such people take large doses of vitamin C, they may experience an accumulation in the kidneys of one of the waste by-products of the vitamin, oxalic acid, which may promote the formation of kidney stones. The possibility also exists that gout—a very painful inflammation of the joints—may be triggered or intensified by high concentrations of vitamin C. Gout is caused by the formation of uric-acid crystals in the joints, and anything that changes the acid balance in the body—as the acidic vitamin C sometimes does—could affect the ailment.

Also of concern is the possibility that huge vitamin C doses will have adverse interactions with other drugs. One conflict frequently cited in medical literature is with warfarin, used to prevent and treat clots in blood vessels. Large amounts of vitamin C may cause warfarin to pass through the digestive system faster than it can be absorbed into the bloodstream. Large quantities of vitamin C may also cause some antidepressants and energizing drugs to be excreted more rapidly, cutting short their desired effect. Extra vitamin C might also distort the results of the urine-sugar tests routinely taken by some diabetics, giving the patient false information on which to determine his insulin dosage. (It was formerly believed that vitamin C slowed down the body's excretion of aspirin, posing the risk of dangerous accumulations of this frequently used drug. But clinical studies in the late 1970s reduced that concern, at least, for those taking up to 3,000 milligrams of vitamin C per day.)

Diarrhea and intestinal discomfort are the most common side effects of heavy vitamin C dosage. Blood-clotting problems and vitamin C dependency followed by withdrawal reactions are still other potential side effects about which there is much speculation but little knowledge. Until such information is developed—and until you are assured that none of these dangers apply to you—it seems reasonable to accept the medical consensus: Get your vitamin C in normal quantities from a balanced diet, and do not attempt to forestall or cure colds with extra-large doses.

## A man-made substance that could prevent colds

The lack of enthusiasm for vitamin C among scientists seeking a cold cure is balanced by their hopes for several other biological and synthetic chemicals that have the potential to block viral reproduction or spread. Among these substances, interferon is perhaps the most promising.

Interferon was discovered in 1957 by the British virologist Alick Isaacs and his Swiss colleague, Jean Lindenmann. Through a chance conversation at London's National Institute for Medical Research, the two specialists discovered that they shared a mutual fascination with a scarcely understood phenomenon known as viral interference: Victims of one kind of viral disease seemingly became immune at the same time to any other viral disease, even when they were exposed to potent viruses. The two scientists joined forces for a series of experiments in which they infected membrane cells in chicken eggs with influenza viruses and then added a second batch of a different virus to the culture. True to expectations, the originally infected cells proved invulnerable to the second wave of attackers.

Delving further, Isaacs and Lindenmann identified the interfering agent as a substance produced in minute quantities by cells that have been infected by a virus. This agent prevents viruses reproduced within an infected cell from taking over nearby healthy cells and spreading further.

As the victim cell begins making duplicate viruses under orders from the invader, it also begins setting up a resistance movement in the form of this mysterious substance, which Isaacs and Lindenmann named interferon. The interferon is released into fluid surrounding the infected cell, where it apparently acts as an intercellular alarm, alerting potential victim cells to impending attack. The warning—which takes place when the interferon makes contact with receptors in the walls of these as yet healthy cells—triggers the production of antiviral proteins, or AVPs. These substances, working in ways not fully understood, ultimately provide protection, preventing the cell from submitting to the orders of the original virus's offspring. Most important, the AVPs set off a general alert, blocking the effects of not only the original viral type but also of virtually any other virus circulating in the system at the time.

This marvelous broad-spectrum protective mechanism, researchers have found, begins to work within several hours after the initial viral invasion. The amount of interferon produced is usually insufficient to block all of the viruses before infection takes some toll in damaged and destroyed cells. But the substance is critical in slowing viral spread, thereby buying the body time to mount its other defenses—eater

cells, killer T cells and so on—in a combined effort to terminate infection.

The effectiveness of interferon against colds was demonstrated in 1973 by Dr. Thomas Merigan of Stanford University and a group of researchers at Britain's Common Cold Unit. They tested it on groups of volunteers who were deliberately exposed to the common rhino type of cold virus. Five of the 16 subjects who received no interferon showed significant symptoms of infection following exposure to cold viruses; none of the 16 volunteers receiving interferon showed any symptoms. This landmark experiment showed for the first time that interferon applied artificially could block viral reproduction and spread in a human respiratory infection. It

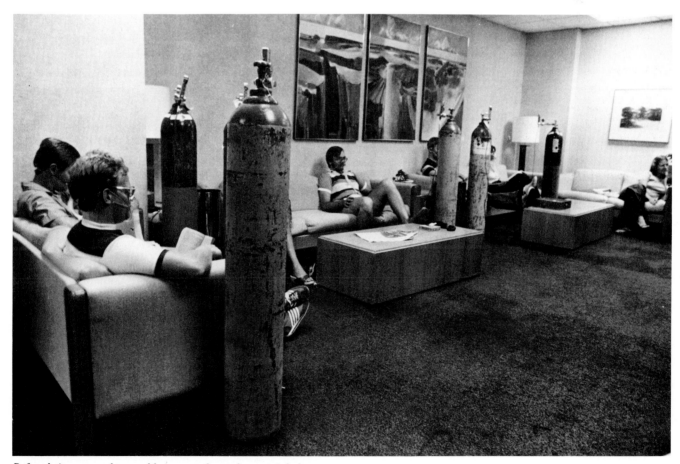

*Before being exposed to a cold virus, student volunteers inhale air dosed with interferon. This part of tests at Baylor and Texas A&M medical schools yielded encouraging results. Less than a third of the students given interferon developed colds, compared with more than half the subjects who did not get interferon.*

was also the first demonstration in history of successful local antiviral treatment for a respiratory infection.

Other similar studies of interferon's power as a cold preventive were begun in 1979 with very small samples of students at the Baylor College of Medicine and Texas A&M University *(page 147)*. In these tests the interferon was administered nasally through an apparatus that produced an aerosol mist. (A control group of volunteers was administered a salt-water aerosol.) The incidence of colds was reduced by almost half in the subjects given interferon.

Interferon, unfortunately, is not only scarce but different in every creature. Unlike antibodies, which can be taken from animals to make human vaccines, interferon from most animals has virtually no effect in humans. Thus, over the initial years of experimentation with this substance, researchers were obliged to depend upon extracts collected with great difficulty from human blood supplies. It takes some 90,000 pints of blood—as much as is donated in Seattle, Washington, in an entire year—to produce 10,000 pints of the crude material from which .014 ounce of interferon can be refined. And because the method of extraction is technically difficult, the supplying of interferon to researchers has been expensive and slow.

The cost of the interferon used in the Common Cold Unit experiment—administered as a nasal spray—was nearly $3,000 per subject tested. Promising though the test results were for progress against colds, Merigan and others experimenting with interferon turned their attention to the substance's value in combating chronic and life-threatening diseases associated with the immune system such as chronic hepatitis, rabies and cancer.

Cold sufferers, however, need not give up on interferon, for a great deal is being done to get around its scarcity and lower its cost. Three strategies are in the experimental stage. It may be possible to find artificial substances that mimic the effects of interferon. When scientists learn more about the nature of a cell's interferon receptors and the internal mechanisms that take direction from them, they may be able to create a compound that, like interferon, will switch on a healthy cell's receptors and make it produce antiviral pro-

teins. Or the antiviral proteins themselves may be synthesized or imitated.

More productive has been a second approach: the creation of agents known as interferon inducers. They are substances that stimulate the body to make extra amounts of its own interferon—but in the absence of infection. Several such inducers have been found as a result of a deeper understanding of the natural actions of the immune system.

The cell's natural production of interferon, it turns out, is stimulated by the internal components of a virus, the nucleic-acid compounds that make up the virus's heredity-controlling ribonucleic and deoxyribonucleic acids—RNA and DNA. In the late 1960s scientists at the Merck Institute for Therapeutic Research in West Point, Pennsylvania, synthesized an RNA-like molecule that proved to be a very potent inducer of interferon production in the test tube, and in animals and humans as well. However, this synthetic, which they named poly I:C, turned out to have some dangerous side effects. So, unfortunately, did several other synthetics with similar powers.

Another promising strategy for making the body produce interferon also involves inducers, but in compounds derived from natural rather than synthetic sources. These so-called biological inducers act like viruses in stimulating interferon production but lack viruses' virulence and contagion. One is endotoxin, a substance in bacterial cell walls that has been found to stimulate interferon production in many types of animal cells. Endotoxin also is poisonous, but some less harmful bacterial product artificially seeded in the respiratory tract of a human cold sufferer could set off a release of booster doses of interferon and antiviral proteins. Similar promise as a biological inducer is shown by the mycoplasmas, cells that resemble—but are smaller than—bacteria.

But the likeliest route to cheap and plentiful interferon seems to lie on the frontiers of genetic engineering in the controversial field known as recombinant DNA technology, or gene splicing. It offers a way to make pure human interferon in vats, milking the priceless elixir from specially bred bacteria. This goal was achieved experimentally in 1979, when a group of scientists led by Dr. Charles Weissmann,

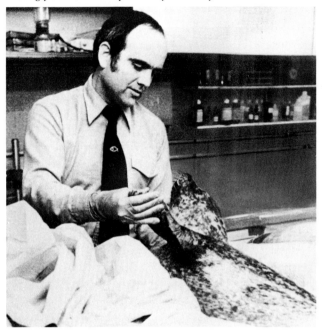

*Investigating the possibility that mammals—including humans —may be susceptible to flu viruses from birds or other nonmammals, a Boston biologist examines one of the hundreds of seals that died of influenza-related pneumonia in New England coastal waters during 1979 and 1980. The seal-epidemic virus is strikingly similar to one previously seen only in birds.*

Professor of Molecular Biology at the University of Zurich, succeeded in synthesizing human interferon outside the body, using something other than human cells.

The scientists isolated the group of nucleic acids—the gene—in human DNA that is responsible for producing interferon in the human body. In a delicate process of biological cut-and-paste, they then spliced this portion of human DNA into the DNA molecule of *Escherichia coli,* a common species of bacteria found in the intestines. The subtly modified *Escherichia coli* grows readily in culture mediums, its recombined DNA molecule producing a protein essentially like human interferon. Though differing somewhat in molecular make-up from interferon, the laboratory product possesses many of the genetic original's antiviral characteristics.

Even in its imperfect state, gene-spliced interferon seems to have a number of major advantages over its current natural and induced counterparts. Once in production, it will be a good deal less expensive than interferon extracted from human blood (*Escherichia coli* is cheap labor). It is also safer

than induced interferon, because no foreign catalyst comes into play. And it can be manufactured on what amounts to an industrial assembly line, in large quantities.

## New drugs that make viruses go away

Interferon has received so much international celebrity that significant developments in another kind of cure for respiratory infection—synthetic chemical compounds that would kill viruses the way antibiotics kill bacteria—have gone almost unnoticed. None is yet effective against colds, but one such chemical, given the generic name amantadine hydrochloride and the trade name Symmetrel by its makers, E. I. du Pont de Nemours & Co., not only has gone through the long stages of laboratory experiment and clinical testing, but has actually reached the market as a prescription drug for influenza A. Amantadine is a molecule with an unusually symmetrical shape, resembling a diamond. Through mechanisms not yet identified, amantadine keeps the influenza-A virus from initiating new growth in the respiratory tract. Whether taken as a preventive before the onset of flu symptoms or as a treatment afterward, it quickly goes to work either blocking penetration of the virus into healthy cells or inhibiting some early phase of viral replication in those cells.

Amantadine's journey from the test tube to the drugstore shows the obstacles that must be overcome by any new drug but particularly by one designed for respiratory infections. Amantadine emerged from the standard drug-company technique of screening promising compounds to find one or two that showed potential against a chosen target—in this case respiratory viruses. Then the researchers synthesized related compounds and tried them. One, amantadine, proved highly effective against influenza A. It then underwent years of trials in animals to see what desirable and undesirable effects it produced and to set preliminary dosage levels that could be applied to humans. At that point, Du Pont secured government permission to test it on humans as what the U.S. Food and Drug Administration calls an investigational new drug.

In 1963 a University of Illinois team headed by Dr. George Gee Jackson, one of the leading figures in respiratory-disease research, demonstrated that amantadine produced up to a 70 per cent reduction in clinical illness from influenza A. After several more years of testing the drug for safety and efficacy, Du Pont applied for permission to market it.

Because knowledge of the idiosyncratic nature of influenza viruses is so hazy, only a limited license for amantadine's use was granted. The drug could be sold to treat but one strain of flu, Asian H2N2, the strain used in tests and prevalent in the general population in the early 1960s. Then, shortly after the license was issued in 1966, an event occurred that was to give the rapidly advancing amantadine a serious setback. The existing influenza-A strain went through a major shift—a new strain called A/Hong Kong/68 (H3N2) swept the world.

Without satisfying official requirements for further clinical trials involving the Hong Kong strain but with laboratory evidence on its side, Du Pont urged doctors to use amanta-dine as a preventive against the new influenza-A strain. This action proved a major legal and tactical error, for the company was ordered to retract its statements in a letter sent to every physician in the United States. As far as flu sufferers were concerned, no antiviral drug was available in 1969.

Amantadine simultaneously ran into trouble with some medical authorities, who believed that viruses, being natural parasites of humans, were so intimately involved with the life processes of human cells that they could not be selectively destroyed or inhibited by any drug, amantadine included. To attack the virus, these critics asserted, was to attack the cell, with consequences of a potentially very serious nature.

In the face of worsening publicity and legal obstacles, amantadine might have been withdrawn from production in the United States, even though Du Pont had already spent

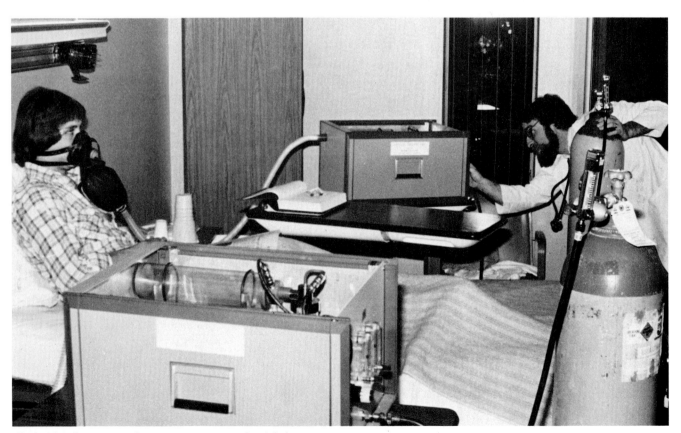

*Abed with influenza, a student uses an oxygen mask to inhale ribavirin, an experimental antiviral drug, while a doctor adjusts a unit that mixes ribavirin and air into a fine mist. (A similar device is seen in the foreground.) In early tests ribavirin—one of several cold or flu fighters under study at the Baylor College of Medicine (page 147)—eased the body aches and fever of flu.*

millions of dollars in carrying it from invention to this stalemate. But an 11th-hour discovery that amantadine had another, quite unrelated, use kept it on the market. A woman suffering from the degenerative nervous disorder called Parkinson's disease was told by her doctor to take amantadine as a flu preventive—and found to her astonishment that the Parkinsonian tremors and loss of movement were markedly alleviated. Doctors traced the serendipitous effects to amantadine, and it came into widespread use for this ailment over the next several years. As a result, many lingering questions as to its possible toxicity were favorably answered.

As had been claimed all along, amantadine turned out to be extremely selective—it attacked only viruses, and cell function was not tampered with. Its side effects were chiefly mild transitory changes in the function of the central nervous system—lightheadedness, nervousness, difficulty in concentration, insomnia or, contrarily, drowsiness—that occurred in some 7 per cent of users. Such side effects were similar to those sometimes associated with common over-the-counter antihistamines or decongestants.

Reassured by these findings and by reports from Europe, particularly from the Soviet Union, of amantadine's value in treating a number of influenza-A strains, the United States formally licensed amantadine's broader use in 1976. Today, amantadine is recommended for prevention of influenza A (but not for influenza B or any other respiratory virus). It also can be used to treat an existing influenza-A infection—particularly within the first 48 hours after symptoms appear—but with less efficacy than as a preventive.

Amantadine is not suggested as an equal alternative to vaccination. To protect yourself against influenza, you are still advised to follow your physician's judgment on whether or not you fall into one of the risk groups and should receive a shot. Rather, amantadine is best used along with other strategies for controlling flu, particularly during epidemics.

Amantadine can protect individuals while they develop maximum immunity following vaccination. Amantadine is also the only alternative for individuals who for some reason cannot tolerate flu vaccines—for example, people who are allergic to eggs, in which the vaccines are grown. It may also be an effective reinforcer of immunity for those who have been vaccinated but fall into the high-risk category—hospital patients, the chronically ill, and people in semiclosed communities, particularly members of that double-jeopardy group, the elderly in old-age homes.

Where prevention is the goal, the recommended adult dosage of amantadine is 100 milligrams twice a day for 30 to 60 days, the usual span of a local flu epidemic, or for the two weeks or so required for a vaccination to take full effect. Therapeutic dosages are also 100 milligrams twice a day, beginning, if possible, within 48 hours after the onset of symptoms and continuing for up to two days after the last sign of illness disappears, usually about a week later. While amantadine as a therapeutic cannot abruptly terminate the infection, it does have some effect in reducing the severity of symptoms, possibly reducing in turn the likelihood of those secondary complications, such as pneumonia, that add so greatly to flu's potential dangers. Amantadine also seems to bring about a significant reduction in the amount of flu virus a carrier sheds, an effect that helps contain the infection once it gets within the precincts of the family.

Now that amantadine has successfully blazed a trail, many more antiviral drugs seem certain to follow. Rimantadine, closely related to amantadine but lacking some of its side effects, is currently under study in the United States and is already being used against influenza A in the Soviet Union, where much research on it has been done. Other compounds having antiviral effects on the herpes simplex virus (which causes cold sores and may be associated with some cancers) have shown promising results in early testing. And at Texas A&M University, student volunteers suffering from flu were given a new experimental drug called ribavirin. According to the study director, Dr. Vernon Knight of the Baylor College of Medicine, ribavirin seemed to alleviate the symptoms of the flu sufferers and showed no toxic effects.

Virtually every large pharmaceutical company in the world has some portion of its research budget invested in the high-stakes race to find a drug to combat cold and flu viruses. For the moment, chicken soup may still be the drug of choice, but more effective help is on the way. ✺

# A virus-ridden vacation at a research laboratory

On the morning of July 29, 1980, John and Pat Lloyd, a Worcester couple, embarked on an odd and, at first glance, somewhat disquieting holiday. To serve in the long, frustrating campaign against the common cold, they checked into a cluster of World War II Quonset huts near Salisbury, England, 90 miles southwest of London — and set out to catch a virus infection.

To the Lloyds, the prospect of becoming volunteers was idyllic; they were, in fact, making their third visit to the Salisbury headquarters of Britain's Common Cold Unit. Fed and lodged at government expense, they could read, fish, ramble through the beautiful countryside, or play badminton, quoits or table tennis. They ran only a 1-in-3 chance of getting sick. Even if they did, their illness would be milder than a normal cold, since the potency of the test viruses is artificially reduced. And the unit's isolation procedure, which requires volunteers to stay at least 30 feet away from everyone but their roommates, is a boon to most volunteers: It creates the luxury of complete privacy.

For all its holiday air, however, the Common Cold Unit is a serious scientific establishment, one of the most renowned virus research centers in the world. Since its founding in 1946, the unit has done pioneering research into virtually every aspect of the common cold: how people transmit and contract cold viruses, how antibodies protect against colds, and how human viruses and antibodies behave in the laboratory.

Today the unit has shifted its primary attention to influenza, a more serious respiratory ailment. But its methods remain the same. Human subjects are necessary, for the only animals that catch truly human colds are scarce and uncooperative chimpanzees. Every two weeks, about 30 men and women come for a 10-day visit and, in the interest of science, do their best to get sick.

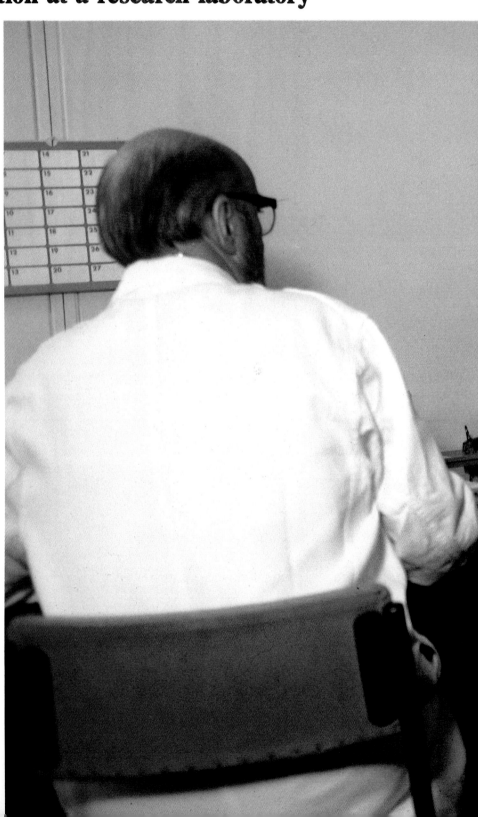

*Upon their arrival at the Common Cold Unit, John and Pat Lloyd are examined by the clinical director, Dr. John Wallace. He screens out volunteers who have suffered such ailments as tuberculosis, asthma, hay fever, sinusitis or drug allergies, which might risk complications during the experiment, and makes sure that potential subjects do not already have incipient colds.*

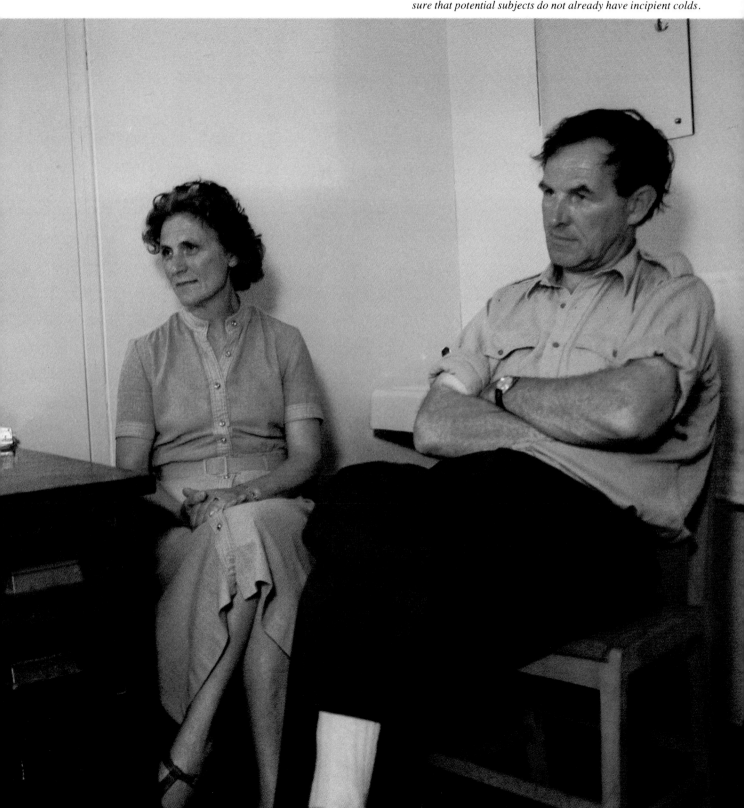

154

# Catering to avoid contamination

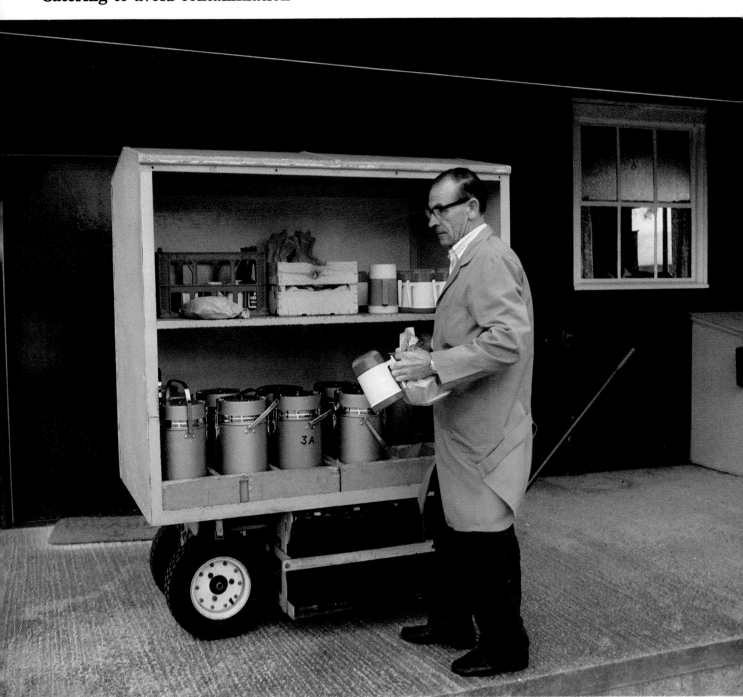

*As the Lloyds peer through their window, a deliveryman
arrives with a battery-driven cart carrying hot midday meals. To
be sure that viruses are not transmitted from couple to couple
through the food, each five-room vacation flat has its own set of
insulated containers, clearly marked to avoid mix-ups.*

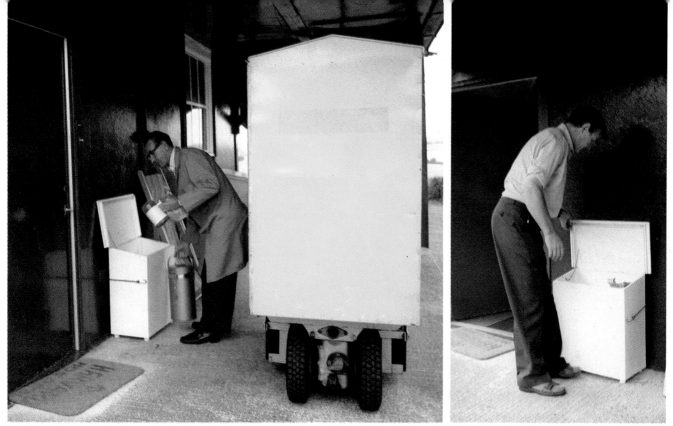

*The deliveryman deposits the Lloyds' lunch (left), then rings the doorbell; John Lloyd must wait for him to leave before taking the food inside.*

*The Lloyds share a meal of beef stew. After they wash the pots and put them outside to be picked up, they can leave their flat for recreation.*

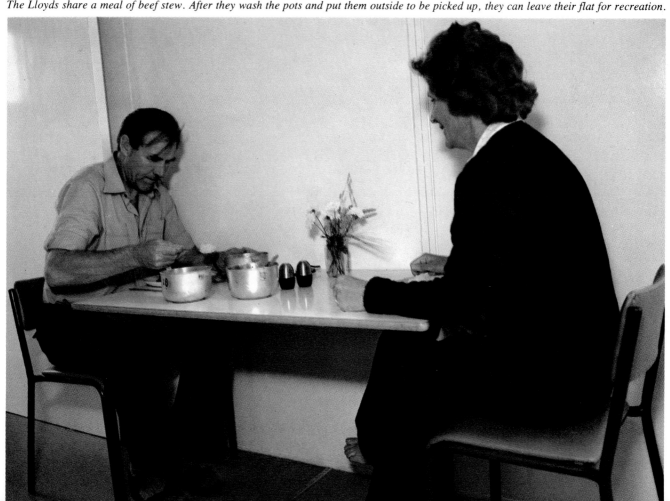

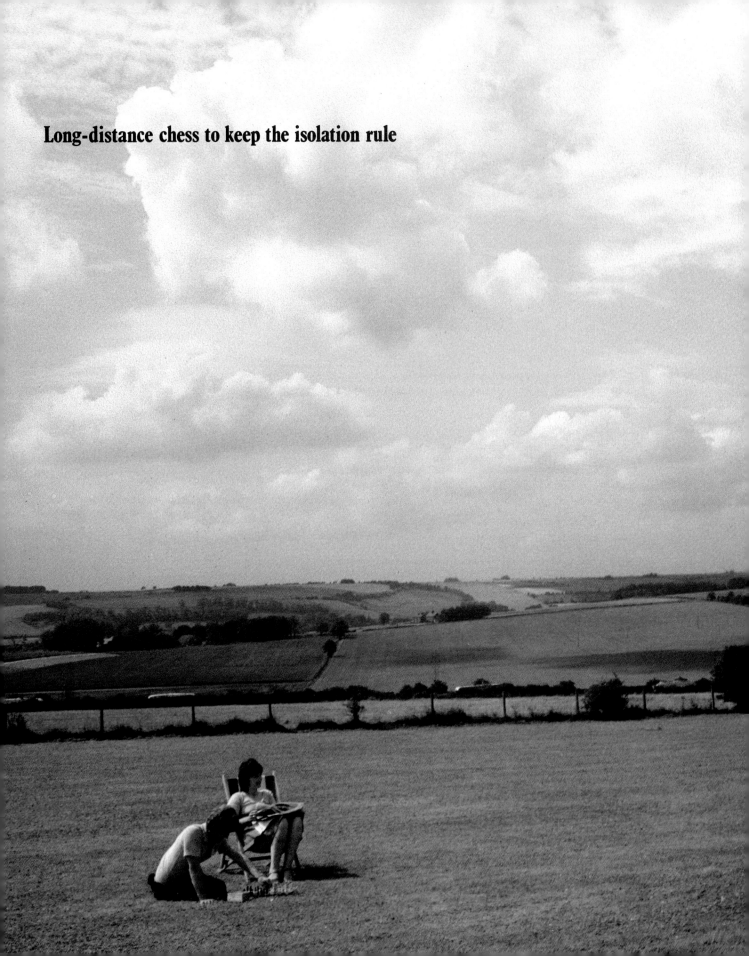

Long-distance chess to keep the isolation rule

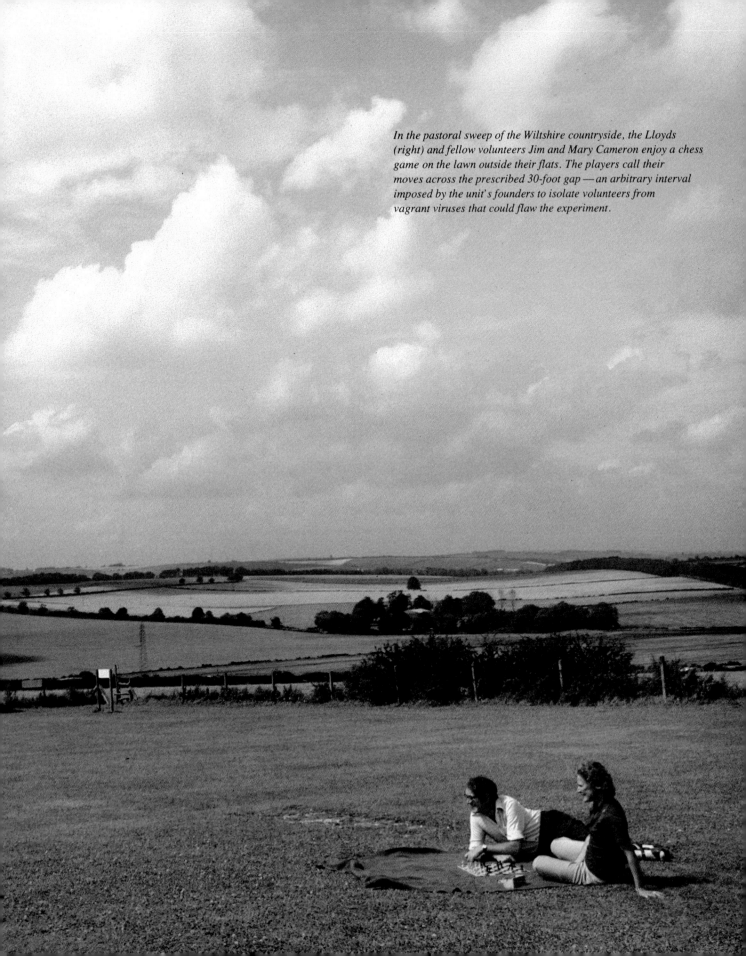

*In the pastoral sweep of the Wiltshire countryside, the Lloyds (right) and fellow volunteers Jim and Mary Cameron enjoy a chess game on the lawn outside their flats. The players call their moves across the prescribed 30-foot gap — an arbitrary interval imposed by the unit's founders to isolate volunteers from vagrant viruses that could flaw the experiment.*

158

# Check-ups that establish norms for a test

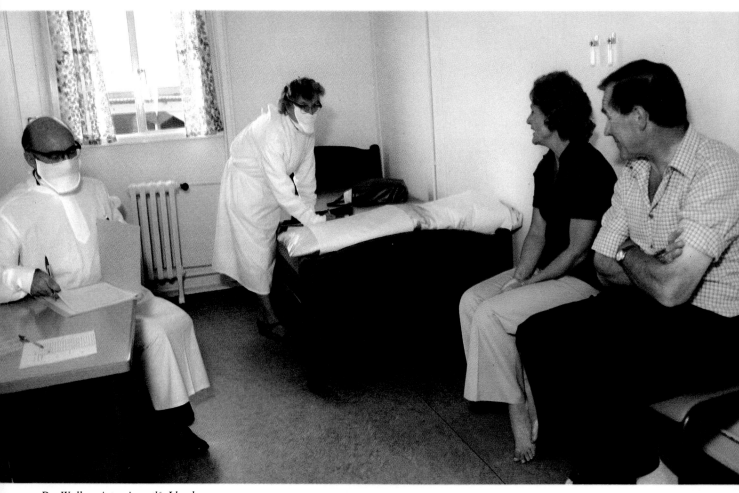

Dr. Wallace interviews the Lloyds
in their flat while a matron records their
temperatures from a chart they fill in
morning and night. The masks are designed
not so much to protect the staff as to
avoid infecting volunteers with stray viruses.

To be sure Pat is not coming down with a
cold, Dr. Wallace examines her throat. His
data on the usual health of the volunteers
serve as a base line to verify whether they
are infected by the experimental virus.

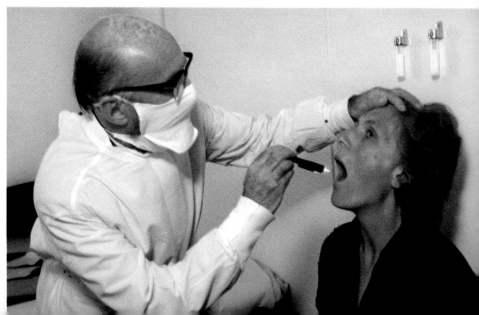

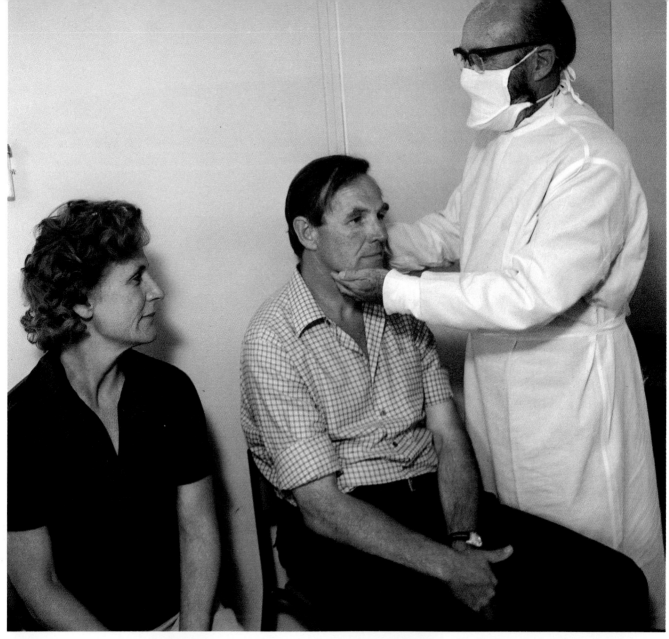

*Dr. Wallace checks John's adenoid glands, applying pressure through the neck. He has already determined the glands' normal size and is now trying to detect any swelling in them—one of the early symptoms of a virus infection.*

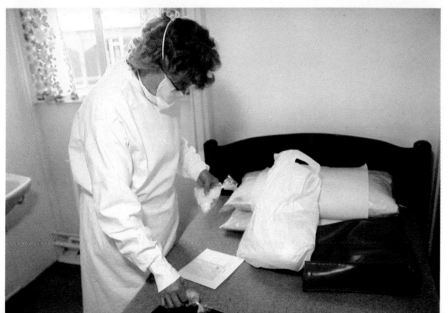

*To gauge the normal amounts of nasal secretion for later comparison, the matron counts the Lloyds' used tissues, which have been stored in individual cellophane bags for the daily inspection.*

260

# Trying to catch flu—scientifically

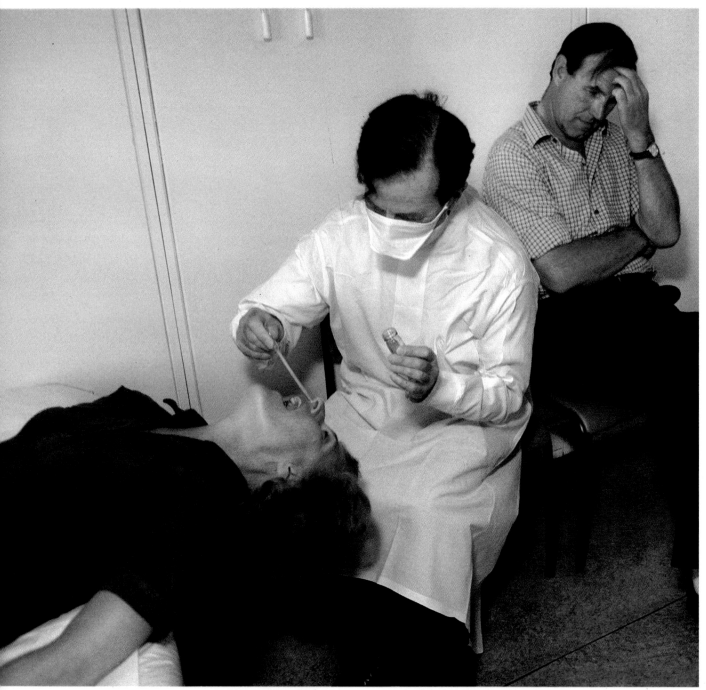

*The Cold Unit's virologist, Dr. A. S. Beare, administers nose*
*drops to Pat Lloyd. John received a dose of the same drops, which*
*contain a strain of bird influenza for an experiment testing*
*the theory that humans can be infected by animal flu viruses. Dr.*
*Beare is the only person who knows which subjects receive live*
*viruses and which ones receive a harmless substitute, or placebo.*

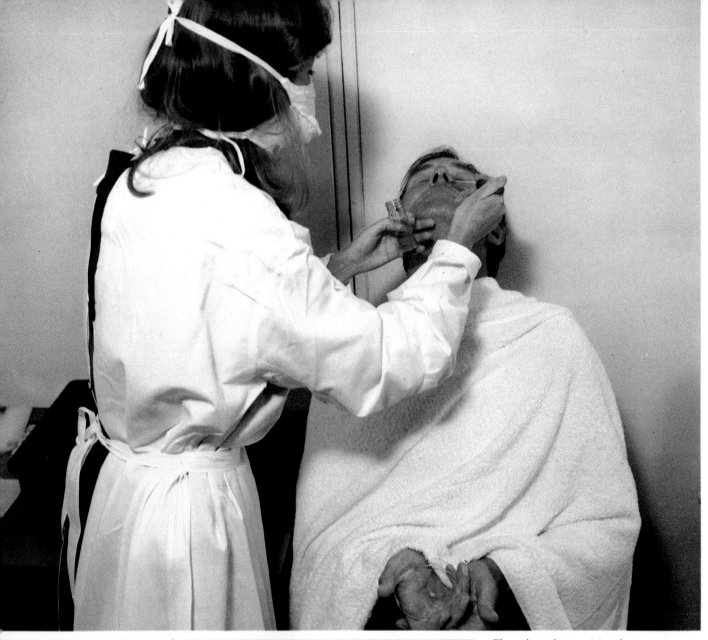

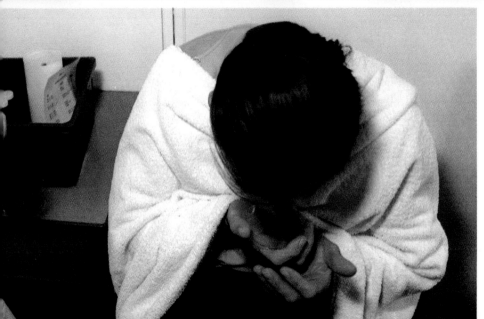

Three days after receiving the virus, John is given a nasal washing. A laboratory technician drops a mild salt solution into his nose (above), then he bends forward so that the solution drips into a plastic dish (left). Although both John and Pat felt slightly unwell, a laboratory analysis of the solution found no virus in it. Blood tests taken two weeks after they left the unit indicated that they had not developed antibodies to the virus, confirming that they did not in fact catch flu.

# A festive release to the outside world

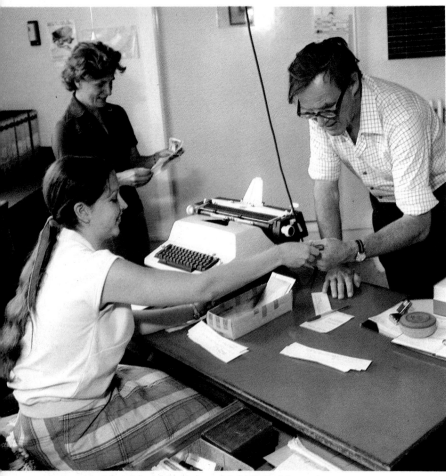

At the end of their stay at the Common Cold Unit, John and
Pat collect their accrued pocket money—£10 apiece—from Dr.
Wallace's secretary. As three-time volunteer subjects, they
also received colorful lapel pins shaped like a cold virus.

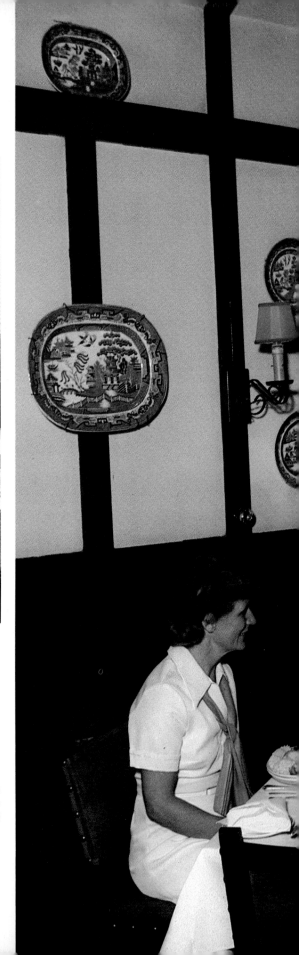

The Lloyds celebrate their return to society by dining in
style at the Red Lion Hotel, a famous landmark in Salisbury. They
feasted on a prime rib roast with all the trimmings — a special
treat after 10 days of nourishing but drab institutional food.

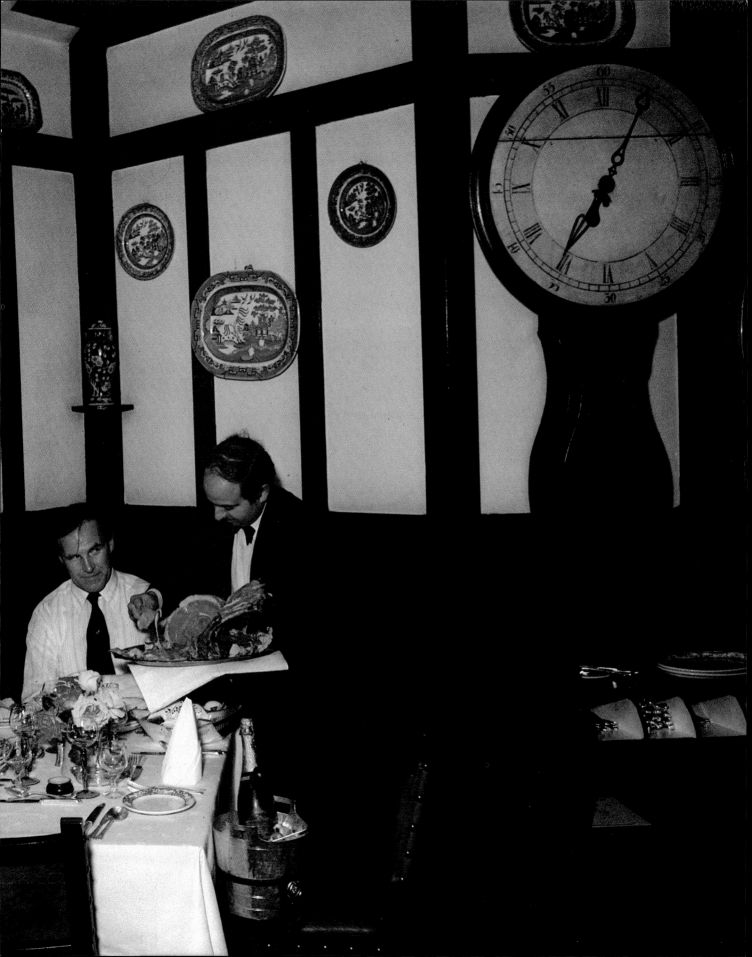

# An encyclopedia of symptoms

*The symptoms of the common cold are familiar discomforts that can be misleading, for they are sometimes also indications of more serious diseases. The ability to recognize the subtle differences between the signals of a cold and those of other diseases can be vital. The most common indications of a cold and of diseases often mistaken for a cold are described below, listed alphabetically by symptoms that can be felt or seen. The disease that causes each symptom—or each group of symptoms—is named in small capital letters.*

**B**ACK PAIN. For mild back pain that is accompanied by the usual cold symptoms, use aspirin and apply heat to the back.

● **Back pain accompanied by leg aches, sore throat, headache, fever and a dry cough** may be a sign of INFLUENZA. If the fever rises above 102° F., if the cough becomes severe or productive, or if you are elderly or have a chronic ailment, consult a physician.

**BREATHING DIFFICULTY.** Breathing difficulty can arise not only from respiratory infections but also from causes as diverse as lung damage, heart disease and cancer.

● **Breathing difficulty produced by a stuffy, runny nose** is a basic symptom of a COLD. No medical treatment is necessary, but you may get temporary relief by using a vaporizer, drinking liquids and taking a decongestant.

● **Shortness of breath accompanied by chest pain, fever and a cough that produces mucus** is a symptom of BRONCHITIS, a bacterial or viral infection of the bronchial tubes. If the symptoms are severe or persist longer than 10 days, consult a physician.

● **Breathing difficulty in children** who have other symptoms beyond those of a cold can indicate any of three serious diseases.

*If a child breathes with a croaking sound, is hoarse and has a barking cough* with choking spasms, the symptoms may indicate CROUP, a viral or bacterial infection of the larynx and lower respiratory tract. The child's small airway may be blocked by the rapid swelling of the larynx, presenting a danger of suffocation. Moist air may help open the airway until a choking spasm subsides; take the child to the bathroom immediately, turn on a hot water tap full force and close the bathroom door to trap the steam. Keep the child calm and consult a physician as soon as possible. If the child's breathing has not improved after 10 minutes or so, take him to the nearest hospital emergency room for treatment.

*If a child has breathing difficulty accompanied by fever, headache, swallowing difficulty, severe sore throat, nausea and vomiting,* he may have DIPHTHERIA, a bacterial infection of the throat. Consult a physician immediately.

*If a child's breathing difficulty follows violent coughing* (some-times eight to 10 coughs in a single breath), the cause may be WHOOPING COUGH, a bacterial infection that generally strikes children under the age of two. The disease may start with typical cold symptoms such as sneezing, a runny, stuffed-up nose, and general listlessness; later symptoms may include a bluish face and vomiting. Consult a physician for treatment.

● **Breathing difficulty accompanied by chest pain,** fever, headache and a painful cough that produces yellow, pink or rust-colored mucus may indicate PNEUMONIA, a bacterial or viral infection of the lungs. Consult a physician immediately.

● **Breathing difficulty accompanied by nausea and vomiting, sore throat, neck and joint stiffness,** fever, headache, and swallowing difficulty may be caused by POLIOMYELITIS, a viral infection of the nervous system. Consult a physician immediately.

● **Periodic breathing difficulty accompanied by a feeling of tightness in the chest,** a cough and wheezing may signal an allergic disease, BRONCHIAL ASTHMA. Consult a physician for treatment.

● **Shortness of breath without exertion,** an enlarged, barrel-like chest and spasmodic attacks of coughing that produce thick mucus are possible signs of PULMONARY EMPHYSEMA, a disease marked by damaged lung tissue. Consult a physician as soon as possible.

**C**HILLS. *See FEVER*

**COUGH.** Coughing protects the lower respiratory tract from invasion by particles and mucus, but all coughs are irritating, and some may be symptoms of a serious infection or disorder.

There are two basic types of coughs. A cough that brings up mucus, a productive cough, protects the lungs from further damage from infection. Do not use medicines to suppress this kind of cough. A nonproductive, or dry, cough usually results from irritation caused by mucus dripping from the nasal passages to the throat. Nonproductive coughs may be eased by sucking on hard candy or lozenges or by cough suppressants available without prescription. Aspirin or acetaminophen, pain-killing medications found in some lozenges, may also reduce sensitivity to the irritation.

Both types of cough can be soothed by thinning the mucus secreted during a respiratory infection. Drink plenty of liquids and increase the moisture in the air with a vaporizer.

● **A nonproductive cough with a stuffed-up, runny nose, sneezing and sore throat** is a classic symptom of a common COLD.

*If a nonproductive cough is associated with back and leg aches,* sore throat, fever and headache, you may have INFLUENZA. If the fever rises above 102° F. in an adult or 103° F. in a child, if the cough becomes severe or productive, or if you are elderly or have a chronic lung or heart ailment, consult a physician for treatment.

● **A productive cough** accompanied by the symptoms listed above may occasionally be a sign of a cold or flu. Different or additional symptoms, however, may indicate a more serious origin.

*If a productive cough occurs with chest pain, fever and breathing difficulty,* you may have BRONCHITIS, a bacterial or viral infection of the bronchial tubes. Consult a physician if the symptoms are severe or persist beyond 10 days.

*If a cough produces yellow, pink or rust-colored mucus and is accompanied by chest pains,* breathing difficulty, fever and headache, you may have PNEUMONIA, a bacterial or viral infection of the lungs. Consult a physician as soon as possible.

*If violent coughs (sometimes eight to 10 times in one breath) are followed by gasping for air,* the cause may be WHOOPING COUGH, a bacterial infection that generally strikes children under the age of two. The disease may start with cold symptoms such as sneezing, a runny, stuffed-up nose, and listlessness. Other symptoms include a bluish face and vomiting. Consult a physician for treatment.

*If a hacking cough is accompanied by a pink rash,* fever, red eyes and muscle pain, the cause may be one of two related viral diseases, MEASLES or GERMAN MEASLES. Both are more common in children than in adults. Isolate the sufferer and consult a physician. A pregnant woman who has been exposed to German measles should consult a physician immediately.

*If a periodic cough is accompanied by wheezing, breathing difficulty and a feeling of tightness in the chest,* you may have BRONCHIAL ASTHMA, an allergy. Consult a physician for treatment.

*If a periodic productive cough is accompanied by constant breathing difficulty and the development of an enlarged, barrel-like chest,* the cause may be PULMONARY EMPHYSEMA, or damaged lung tissue. Consult a physician as soon as possible.

*If a chronic cough produces thick mucus and occurs with fatigue,* you may have TUBERCULOSIS, a bacterial infection of the lungs. Consult a physician immediately.

**D**IZZINESS. Dizziness during or shortly after a cold may be caused by ear infections. It may also result from the use of alcohol, sedatives or certain cold medicines, or from more serious disorders such as brain damage. If dizziness is severe and does not accompany or follow an upper respiratory infection, consult a physician.

● **Dizziness accompanied by earache, a feeling of fullness or ringing in the ears, fever and occasionally loss of hearing** may be caused by OTITIS MEDIA, a bacterial or viral infection of the middle ear. This complication of a cold is more common in children than in adults. Consult a physician for treatment.

**DRY THROAT.** *See TICKLE IN THE THROAT*

**E**ARACHE. Earache may be a direct symptom of a cold, or may result from a bacterial infection accompanying or following a cold. Any earache requires a physician's examination. A warm, moistened towel or a heating pad applied to the ear may offer some comfort until a doctor can be seen; aspirin or acetaminophen may also help relieve pain temporarily. Do not plug your ear with cotton swabs or insert sharp objects in your ear.

● **An earache associated with fever, loss of hearing, dizziness and a fullness or ringing in the ear** may be caused by OTITIS MEDIA, a bacterial or viral complication of a cold, more common in children than in adults. Consult a physician as soon as possible.

EYE WATERING. Watery eyes are a common symptom of respiratory ailments, but may also result from simple irritation, or from more serious conditions such as CONJUNCTIVITIS.

● **Watery eyes accompanied by a stuffed-up, runny nose, breathing difficulty, sore throat, coughing and sneezing** are generally caused by a cold. The secretions will end with the infection. For temporary relief bathe the eyes with warm water or eyedrops; if symptoms are severe or affect vision, consult a physician.

● **Watery eyes that become red and itchy or are sealed shut in the morning by a puslike discharge** may be caused by CONJUNCTIVITIS, a viral or bacterial infection of the mucous membrane that lines the inner surface of the eyelids. Consult a physician.

**F**ATIGUE. A general feeling of tiredness, usually accompanying a fever, is a fairly common symptom of respiratory infections. Many medications will also make you feel tired. If you frequently feel tired without any clear reason, consult a physician.

● **Extreme fatigue** that prevents you from carrying on your everyday activities may signal either of two serious ailments.

*If you experience extreme fatigue accompanied by swollen glands in the neck and jaws,* general achiness, fever, headache, sore throat and occasionally a rash, you may have INFECTIOUS MONONUCLEOSIS, a viral infection of the lymph nodes and spleen. Consult a physician for a blood test. Bed rest, aspirin or acetaminophen, and a salt-water gargle (one half teaspoon of salt to a cup of warm water) will help relieve discomfort.

*If you experience extreme fatigue accompanied by chest pains,* fever and a chronic cough producing thick mucus, you may have TUBERCULOSIS, a bacterial infection of the lungs. Consult a physician as soon as possible.

FEVER. In children, but seldom in adults, an abnormal rise in body temperature often accompanies such COLD symptoms as a sore throat, coughing, sneezing and a stuffed-up or runny nose. In adults, fever is more common in bacterial infections. Bed rest, aspirin or acetaminophen, and cool baths will usually lower temperature. Increased perspiration during a high fever, particularly in children, may cause dehydration, or loss of body fluids; offer your child small portions of water or fruit juices. If temperature rises above 102° F. in an adult or 103° F. in a child, consult a physician.

● **Fever accompanied by symptoms other than those of a cold** may signal any of a wide variety of diseases.

*If fever is accompanied by back and leg aches,* sore throat, headache and a dry cough, you may have INFLUENZA. If your fever is high, if your cough is severe or productive of mucus, or if you are elderly or have a chronic lung or heart ailment, consult a physician.

*If fever occurs with a cough that produces mucus* and if you have breathing difficulty, chest pain and malaise, you may have BRONCHITIS, a bacterial or viral infection of the bronchial tubes. Consult a physician if symptoms are severe or last beyond 10 days.

*If fever is accompanied by difficulty in swallowing, sore throat, red and swollen tonsils,* and perhaps swollen glands in the neck, you may have TONSILLITIS, a bacterial or viral infection of the tonsils, more common in children than in adults. If the symptoms are severe, consult a physician. Mild symptoms may be relieved with aspirin or acetaminophen, a salt-water gargle (one half teaspoon of salt to a cup of warm water), and small portions of liquids.

*If fever is accompanied by thick white or yellow spots at the back of the throat,* you may have STREP THROAT, a bacterial·infection. Consult a physician to arrange for a throat culture. Strep infections can lead to serious disorders of the heart and kidneys.

*If fever occurs with breathing difficulty, chest pain,* headache and a painful cough that produces yellow, pink or rust-colored mucus, you may have PNEUMONIA, a bacterial or viral infection of the lungs. Consult a physician as soon as possible.

*If fever is accompanied by swollen glands near the ears,* swallowing difficulty and headache, you may have MUMPS, a viral infection of the salivary glands. In children, mumps may be treated by isolating patients and giving them aspirin or acetaminophen, and liquids, but if the symptoms are severe, consult a physician. Males over the age of puberty who are exposed to mumps and have not had them in childhood should consult a physician as soon as possible.

*If fever occurs with headache and a red rash* that generally starts on the trunk and later scabs over, the cause may be CHICKEN POX, a viral infection, more common in children than in adults. Bed rest, aspirin, fluids and treatment of the scabs with calamine lotion or other preparations to relieve itching are effective home treatments.

*If fever occurs with a pink rash, runny nose, cough, red eyes* and muscle pain, the cause may be one of two related viral diseases, MEASLES or GERMAN MEASLES, both more common in children than in adults. Isolate the sufferer and consult a physician. Pregnant women who have been exposed to German measles should consult a physician as soon as possible.

*If fever is accompanied by a reddish body rash,* sore throat, swollen glands in the neck, headache, nausea and vomiting, the cause may be SCARLET FEVER, a bacterial infection that usually attacks children. Consult a physician.

*If fever occurs with extreme fatigue, swollen glands in the neck and jaws,* achiness, headache, sore throat, and perhaps a rash, you may have INFECTIOUS MONONUCLEOSIS, a viral infection of the lymph nodes and spleen. Consult a physician. Bed rest, aspirin or acetaminophen, and a salt-water gargle (one half teaspoon of salt to a cup of warm water) will help relieve discomfort.

*If a child has a fever accompanied by breathing and swallowing difficulty, headache,* severe sore throat, nausea and vomiting, the cause may be DIPHTHERIA, a bacterial infection of the throat. Consult a physician immediately.

*If fever is accompanied by headache, neck stiffness* so severe that touching the chin to the chest is impossible, and changes in consciousness, the cause may be either MENINGITIS, a bacterial or viral infection of the spinal cord, or ENCEPHALITIS, a viral infection of the brain. Consult a physician immediately.

*If fever occurs with swollen, painful joints (usually the knees, wrists and elbows),* general fatigue, and perhaps a rash, you may have RHEUMATIC FEVER, a serious bacterial infection that can damage the heart. Consult a physician immediately.

**H**EADACHE. Headache may be a symptom of a COLD, but it also accompanies a wide range of disorders, from emotional stress to brain damage. A mild headache may be relieved by aspirin or acetaminophen. Frequent or severe headaches and headaches that last longer than 24 hours require medical attention.

● **A headache that occurs with back and leg aches,** sore throat, fever and a dry cough may indicate INFLUENZA. If fever rises above 102° F. in adults or 103° F. in children, if the cough becomes severe or productive, or if you are elderly or suffering from a chronic lung or heart ailment, consult a physician.

● **A headache following a cold, located at the front of the head and accompanied by general achiness** and thick or bloody nasal mucus may be caused by SINUSITIS, a bacterial infection of the sinuses. Mild symptoms may be relieved by taking aspirin or acetaminophen and by applying warm, wet compresses to the forehead or alternating warm and cool compresses. If symptoms are severe or last longer than three weeks, consult a physician.

● **A headache with swollen glands near the ears,** back pain, difficulty in swallowing and fever may be caused by MUMPS, a viral infection of the salivary glands. In children, mumps may be treated by isolating patients and giving them aspirin or acetaminophen, and liquids; if symptoms are severe, consult a physician. Males over the age of puberty who are exposed to mumps and have not had them in childhood should consult a physician as soon as possible.

● **A headache accompanied by fever and a rash that later scabs over** may be caused by CHICKEN POX, a viral infection, more common in children than in adults. Bed rest, aspirin, fluids and treatment of the scabs with calamine lotion or other preparations to relieve itching are effective home treatments.

● **A headache that occurs with a reddish body rash, sore throat,** fever, swollen glands in the neck, nausea and vomiting may be caused by SCARLET FEVER, a bacterial infection that usually attacks children. Consult a physician.

● **A headache accompanied by extreme fatigue, swollen glands in the neck and jaws,** achiness, fever, sore throat and occasionally a rash may indicate INFECTIOUS MONONUCLEOSIS, a viral infection of the lymph nodes and spleen. Consult a physician. Bed rest, aspirin or acetaminophen, and a salt-water gargle (one half teaspoon of salt to a cup of warm water) will help relieve discomfort.

● **A headache that occurs with breathing difficulty, chest pain,** fever and a painful cough that produces yellow, pink or rust-colored mucus may be a symptom of PNEUMONIA, a bacterial or viral infection of the lungs. Consult a physician as soon as possible.

● **A child's headache accompanied by breathing difficulty, fever, swallowing difficulty,** severe sore throat, nausea and vomiting may be caused by DIPHTHERIA, a bacterial infection of the throat. Consult a physician immediately.

● **A headache that occurs with fever,** a neck so stiff that touching the chin to the chest is impossible, and changes in consciousness may be caused by either MENINGITIS, a bacterial or viral infection of the spinal cord, or ENCEPHALITIS, a viral infection of the brain. Consult a physician immediately.

**HOARSENESS.** Hoarseness may be caused by infections of the respiratory tract or may arise from simple irritation of the part of the tract called the larynx, which contains the vocal cords.

● **Occasional hoarseness** after smoking or overusing the voice is a symptom of LARYNGITIS, an inflammation of the mucous membranes of the larynx. Stop smoking and talking; increasing moisture in the air with a vaporizer may also help relieve the condition.

*If a child is hoarse, and has a barking cough and spasms* in which he gasps for breath, he may have CROUP, a viral or bacterial infection of the larynx and lower respiratory tract. For a description and recommendations for treatment, see BREATHING DIFFICULTY.

*If hoarseness continues beyond a month,* you may have growths called CYSTS or POLYPS on the vocal cords or, in a rare instance, CANCER OF THE LARYNX. Consult a physician as soon as possible.

**M**USCLE PAINS. Although muscle pains often accompany respiratory infections, they also, particularly if severe, may indicate disorders ranging from injury to MUSCULAR DYSTROPHY.

● **Muscle pain that is particularly severe in the back and legs** and is accompanied by sore throat, fever, headache and a dry cough may be caused by INFLUENZA. If fever rises above 102° F. in an adult or 103° F. in a child, if the cough becomes severe or productive of mucus, or if you are elderly or suffering from a chronic lung or heart ailment, consult a physician.

*If a child suffers from muscle pain, a pink rash,* runny nose, cough, red eyes and fever, the cause may be one of two related viral diseases, MEASLES or GERMAN MEASLES. Isolate the patient and consult a physician. A pregnant woman who has been exposed to German measles should consult a physician immediately.

**N**AUSEA. Nausea and vomiting are fairly common symptoms of a cold and other respiratory infections, especially among children, but can also signal something as simple as stomach irritation or as serious as stomach poisoning. In a cold, nausea is usually brief; if it continues for several hours, consult a physician. Do not try to eat solid foods, but take liquids to prevent dehydration.

● **Nausea and vomiting in children** may be symptoms of any of three potentially dangerous diseases.

*If nausea in a child occurs with vomiting, a reddish body rash,* sore throat, swollen glands in the neck, and headache, the cause may be SCARLET FEVER, a bacterial infection. Consult a physician.

*If vomiting accompanies violent coughing* (sometimes eight to 10 times in a single breath), followed by gasping for air and a bluish face, the cause may be WHOOPING COUGH, a bacterial infection most common in children under two. The disease may start with typical cold symptoms, such as sneezing, a runny or stuffed-up nose and general listlessness. Consult a physician.

*If a child's nausea and vomiting occur with breathing and swallowing difficulty,* fever, headache and severe sore throat, he may have DIPHTHERIA, a bacterial infection of the throat. Consult a physician immediately.

● **Nausea and vomiting accompanied by breathing difficulty, neck and joint stiffness,** sore throat, fever, headache and swallowing difficulty may be caused by POLIOMYELITIS, a viral infection of the nervous system. Consult a physician immediately.

**NOSE, RUNNING.** An unchecked flow of mucus in the nose may be caused by a respiratory infection or an allergy.

● **A stuffed-up, runny nose accompanied by coughing, sneezing and sore throat** is a classic symptom of a COLD or INFLUENZA. The runny nose helps rid your body of unwanted viruses. Reinforce the process by blowing your nose frequently, but blow gently: Blowing too hard can drive mucus into the sinuses and ears, where it may form a breeding ground for bacterial infection.

*If your runny nose produces thick or bloody mucus after other cold symptoms have vanished,* and you have headaches at the front of the head and general achiness, you may have SINUSITIS, a bacterial infection of the sinuses. Mild symptoms may be relieved by aspirin or acetaminophen and by warm, wet compresses applied to the forehead or alternate warm and cool compresses. If symptoms are severe or last beyond three weeks, consult a physician.

● **A constant or periodic runny nose, especially during the pollen season,** is probably a symptom of an ALLERGY. Antihistamines are effective in reducing allergy symptoms, but if symptoms are severe, consult a physician for treatment.

● **A child's runny nose accompanied by a pink rash, cough, fever, red eyes and muscle pain** may be caused by one of two viral diseases, MEASLES or GERMAN MEASLES. Isolate the patient and consult a physician. A pregnant woman who has been exposed to German measles should consult a physician immediately.

## Ringing in the ears.

**R**INGING IN THE EARS. Ringing in the ears is often associated with ear infections following a COLD in children, but may also be caused by anemia or large doses of aspirin.

● **Ringing in the ears accompanied by earache, a feeling of fullness in the ear,** fever, dizziness and occasionally hearing loss may be due to OTITIS MEDIA, a bacterial or viral infection of the middle ear, arising as a complication of a cold. Consult a physician.

**S**MELL, LOSS OF. A loss of smell is common with nasal congestion caused by an infection. Other causes include obstruction in the nose, damage to the nasal tissues or, rarely, a brain tumor.

The sense of smell is stimulated when particles inhaled from the air and mixed with nasal mucus come into contact with specialized olfactory cells in the upper part of the nose. When the nasal membranes are congested and the air flow over them is reduced or stopped, smelling is weakened or interrupted. Viruses may also directly damage the olfactory cells during an infection.

● **A loss of smell, accompanied by a stuffed-up and runny nose, sneezing, sore throat and coughing,** is probably caused by a COLD. The loss of smell is not serious and will usually end when you are able to breathe normally.

**SNEEZE.** Sneezing, an early symptom of a COLD, occurs when mucous membranes in the nose are irritated. The reflex includes inhaling air, closing the larynx so that air pressure in the lungs is greatly increased, and suddenly reopening the larynx, sending a gush of air out through the nose and mouth. Do not try to suppress a sneeze: The added pressure can drive mucus into the sinuses and ears, where it may form a breeding ground for bacterial infections.

**SORE THROAT.** A sore throat is an inflammation caused by bacterial or viral infection or by irritation. Whatever the cause, you may get some relief by increasing moisture in the air with a vaporizer. Hard candy or throat lozenges will stimulate your salivary glands to moisten your throat, and drinking liquids both soothes the throat and replaces the fluids lost during an infection. You may relieve irritation by gargling with salt water (about one half teaspoon of salt to a cup of warm water), by taking aspirin or acetaminophen, or by sucking lozenges containing local anesthetics. If any sore throat does not improve in five days, consult a physician.

● **A sore throat associated with a stuffed-up or runny nose,** coughing and sneezing is probably caused by a COLD.

● **A sore throat that occurs with aches in the back and legs,** fever, headache and a dry cough is probably due to INFLUENZA. If fever rises above 102° F. in an adult or 103° F. in a child, if the cough becomes severe or productive of mucus, or if you are elderly or have a chronic lung or heart ailment, consult a physician.

● **A sore throat accompanied by symptoms other than those of a cold or influenza** may signal any of a wide variety of diseases.

If a sore throat is accompanied by a cough that produces mucus and by fever and difficult breathing, you may have BRONCHITIS, a bacterial or viral infection of the bronchial tubes. Consult a physician if symptoms are severe or last beyond 10 days.

If a sore throat is accompanied by swallowing difficulty, red, swollen tonsils, fever and perhaps swollen glands in the neck, you may be suffering from TONSILLITIS, a bacterial or viral infection of the tonsils, more common in children than in adults. If the symptoms are so severe that breathing is difficult, consult a physician immediately. Mild symptoms may be relieved by the measures described at the beginning of this entry.

If a sore throat is associated with fever and with thick white or yellow spots at the back of the throat, you may have STREP THROAT, a bacterial infection. Consult a physician for a throat culture. Strep infections can lead to serious disorders of the heart and kidneys.

If a child's sore throat occurs with a reddish body rash, fever, swollen glands in the neck, headache, nausea and vomiting, he may have SCARLET FEVER, a bacterial infection. Isolate the patient and consult a physician.

If a sore throat is accompanied by extreme fatigue, fever, swollen glands in the neck and jaws, achiness, headache and perhaps a rash, the cause may be INFECTIOUS MONONUCLEOSIS, a viral infection of the lymph nodes and spleen. Consult a physician.

If a sore throat occurs with breathing and swallowing difficulty, headache, nausea and vomiting, the cause may be DIPHTHERIA, a bacterial infection. Consult a physician immediately.

If a sore throat is accompanied by breathing and swallowing difficulty, neck and joint stiffness, nausea and vomiting, fever, and headache, you may have POLIOMYELITIS, a viral infection of the central nervous system. Consult a physician immediately.

**STIFF OR SWOLLEN JOINTS.** The achiness that sometimes accompanies a cold and often accompanies influenza does not generally alter the action or appearance of the joints. If your joints stiffen or swell during or after a respiratory infection, watch for additional symptoms that may indicate a serious illness.

● **Swollen, painful joints (usually the knees, wrists and elbows),** fever, general fatigue and perhaps a rash may be caused by RHEUMATIC FEVER, a bacterial infection that can eventually damage the heart. Consult a physician immediately.

● **Stiff joints accompanied by a stiff neck,** nausea and vomiting, sore throat, fever, headache and swallowing difficulty may be caused by POLIOMYELITIS, a viral infection of the nervous system. Consult a physician immediately.

**STUFFED-UP NOSE.** A stuffed-up nose can indicate an allergy or a viral infection of the nasal passages, such as a cold. It is caused by an inflammation of the mucous membranes of the nose.

● **A stuffed-up, runny nose occurring with a cough and sneeze** probably indicates a COLD. Increasing the moisture in the air with a vaporizer may relieve the stuffiness. Decongestant drugs that shrink the mucous membranes also offer temporary relief.

● **Constant or periodic nasal stuffiness, especially during the pollen season,** is probably a sign of an ALLERGY. Antihistamines are generally effective in reducing allergy symptoms, but if the symptoms are severe, consult a physician.

**SWOLLEN GLANDS.** Lymph nodes at the front and sides of the neck and at the underside of the lower jaw often swell in response to respiratory infections, as part of the body's defenses. In other cases, swollen glands may be symptoms of more serious diseases of the blood or of the glands themselves.

● **Swollen glands near the ears accompanied by fever, difficult swallowing,** back pain and headache may be caused by MUMPS, a viral infection of the salivary glands. In children, mumps may be treated by isolating patients and giving them aspirin or acetaminophen, and liquids; if symptoms are severe, consult a physician. Males over the age of puberty who are exposed to mumps and have not had them should consult a physician immediately.

● **Swollen glands in the neck and jaws with extreme fatigue,** fever, general achiness, headache, sore throat and perhaps a rash may be caused by INFECTIOUS MONONUCLEOSIS, a viral infection of the lymph nodes and spleen. Consult a physician. Bed rest, aspirin or acetaminophen, and a salt-water gargle (one half teaspoon of salt to a cup of warm water) will help relieve discomfort.

● **Swollen, tender glands in the neck accompanied by difficult swallowing, red and swollen tonsils,** sore throat and fever may be caused by TONSILLITIS, a bacterial or viral infection of the tonsils, more common in children than in adults. If the symptoms are severe, consult a physician. Mild symptoms may be relieved by aspirin or acetaminophen, a salt-water gargle (one half teaspoon of salt to a cup of warm water) and small, frequent portions of liquid.

● **Swollen glands accompanied by general fatigue and a loss of appetite or weight** may be caused by either LEUKEMIA, cancer of the blood, or HODGKIN'S DISEASE, cancer of the lymph system. Consult a physician immediately.

**T**ASTE, LOSS OF. A partial or complete loss of taste is often associated with viral infections of the upper respiratory tract and the digestive system. It is not generally serious and the sense returns when the infection ends.

Taste is sensed when foods mixed with liquid come in contact with taste buds on the tongue, but the sense of smell is also partially responsible for helping you make taste distinctions. When your mucous membranes are swollen and your nasal passages are plugged by a COLD or an ALLERGY, your ability to smell will be reduced or lost, and your ability to distinguish among flavors will accordingly be impaired.

**THROAT SPOTS. White or yellow spots** at the back of the throat, accompanied by fever and sore throat, may be symptoms of STREP THROAT, an infection of the throat by streptococcus bacteria. Consult a physician to have a throat culture done. Strep infections can lead to serious heart and kidney disorders.

**TICKLE IN THE THROAT.** Tickle in the throat occurs during a COLD when mucus from the nose irritates the throat. It is not serious and usually ends in a few days. Normally your body provides saliva to lubricate the throat. When there is insufficient saliva, your inflamed, irritated throat may become dry. To relieve the tickle, bring moisture to the affected area by drinking liquids or by sucking hard candy or lozenges. Increasing the moisture in the air with a vaporizer may also help.

**V**OMITING. *See NAUSEA*

# Bibliography

## BOOKS

Academy of Traditional Chinese Medicine, *An Outline of Chinese Acupuncture*. Foreign Languages Press, 1975.

Aikman, Lonnelle, *Nature's Healing Arts: From Folk Medicine to Modern Drugs*. National Geographic Society, 1977.

American Medical Association Department of Drugs, *AMA Drug Evaluations*. 4th ed. 1980.

Andrewes, Sir Christopher, *The Common Cold*. Norton, 1965.

Andrewes, Sir Christopher, *In Pursuit of the Common Cold*. Heinemann, 1973.

Beeson, Paul B., *Textbook of Medicine,* Vol. 1. 14th ed. Saunders, 1975.

Bellanti, Joseph A., ed., *Immunology II*. Saunders, 1978.

Benchley, Robert, *From Bed to Worse: Or Comforting Thoughts About the Bison*. Harper, 1934.

Beveridge, W.I.B., *Influenza: The Last Great Plague,* Neale Watson, 1977.

Boston Children's Medical Center and Richard I. Feinbloom, *Child Health Encyclopedia*. Delacorte, 1975.

Bowry, T. R., *Immunology Simplified*. Oxford University Press, 1977.

Brain, Joseph D., Donald F. Proctor, and Lynne M. Reid, eds., *Respiratory Defense Mechanisms*. Marcel Dekker, 1977.

Butterfield, L. H., ed., *Diary and Autobiography of John Adams*. Belknap Press (Harvard University Press), 1961.

Conn, Howard F., ed., *Current Therapy 1967*. Saunders, 1967.

Consumer Guide, *Nonprescription Drugs*. Beekman House, 1979.

Consumer Reports Books, *The Medicine Show*. Pantheon Books, 1980.

Corrigan, L. Luan, ed., *Handbook of Nonprescription Drugs*. American Pharmaceutical Association, 1979.

Crosby, Alfred W., Jr., *Epidemic and Peace, 1918*. Greenwood Press, 1976.

Crouch, James E., *Functional Human Anatomy*. Lea & Febiger, 1972.

Davis, Audrey, and Toby Appel, *Bloodletting Instruments in the National Museum of History and Technology*. Smithsonian Institution Press, 1979.

Di Cyan, Erwin, and Lawrence Hessman, *Without Prescription*. Simon and Schuster, 1972.

Dowling, Harry F., *Fighting Infection*. Harvard University Press, 1977.

Drew, W. Lawrence, *Viral Infections: A Clinical Approach*. Davis, 1976.

Elias, Norbert, *The Civilizing Process*. Urizen Books, 1978.

Evans, Alfred S., ed., *Viral Infections of Humans: Epidemiology and Control*. Plenum, 1976.

Evans, Wayne O., and Jonathan O. Cole, *Your Medicine Chest*. Little, Brown, 1978.

Galasso, George J., Thomas C. Merigan and Robert A. Buchanan, eds., *Antiviral Agents and Viral Diseases of Man*. Raven Press, 1979.

Galton, Lawrence, *The Complete Book of Symptoms and What They Can Mean*. Simon and Schuster, 1978.

Gibbons, Euell, *Stalking the Helpful Herbs*. David McKay, 1970.

Gibbons, Euell, *Stalking the Wild Asparagus*. David McKay, 1962.

Graedon, Joe, and Teresa Graedon, *The People's Pharmacy-2*. Avon Books, 1980.

Grieve, M., *A Modern Herbal*. Dover Publications, 1971.

Guthrie, Helen Andrews, *Introductory Nutrition*. 4th ed. Mosby, 1979.

Hansten, Philip D., *Drug Interactions*. Lea & Febiger, 1979.

Hoehling, A. A., *The Great Epidemic*. Little, Brown, 1961.

Hospital Practice, *Status Report on Influenza*. HP Publishing, 1977.

Imperato, Pascal James, *What to Do About the Flu*. Dutton, 1976.

Jackson, George Gee, and Robert Lee Muldoon, *Viruses Causing Common Respiratory Infections in Man*. University of Chicago Press, 1975.

Kilbourne, Edwin D., ed., *The Influenza Viruses and Influenza*. Academic Press, 1975.

Knight, Vernon, ed., *Viral and Mycoplasmal Infections of the Respiratory Tract*. Lea & Febiger, 1973.

Labaree, Leonard W., ed., *The Papers of Benjamin Franklin*, Vol. 1. Yale University Press, 1959.

Lipton, James M., ed., *Fever*. Raven Press, 1980.

Locke, David, *Viruses: The Smallest Enemy*. Crown Publishers, 1974.

Long, James W., *The Essential Guide to Prescription Drugs*. Harper & Row, 1977.

Lower, Richard, *De Catarrhis 1672*. Dawsons of Pall Mall, 1963.

Miller, Benjamin F., and Claire Brackman Keane, *Encyclopedia and Dictionary of Medicine and Nursing*. Saunders, 1972.

Millspaugh, Charles F., *American Medicinal Plants*. Dover Publications, 1974.

National Research Council, *Recommended Dietary Allowances*. 9th ed. National Academy of Sciences, 1980.

Neustadt, Richard E., and Harvey V. Fineberg, *The Swine Flu Affair*. U.S. Department of Health, Education and Welfare, 1978.

Osborn, June, ed., *Influenza in America 1918-1976: History, Science & Politics*. Neale Watson, 1977.

Pansky, Ben, *Dynamic Anatomy and Physiology*. Macmillan, 1975.

Pauling, Linus, *Vitamin C and the Common Cold*. Freeman, 1970.

*Physicians' Desk Reference for Nonprescription Drugs*. Medical Economics Company, 1980.

Rinzler, Carol Ann, *The Dictionary of Medical Folklore*. Crowell, 1979.

Russell, Francis, *The Great Interlude*. McGraw-Hill, 1964.

Schlossberg, Leon, *The Johns Hopkins Atlas of Human Functional Anatomy*. Johns Hopkins University Press, 1977.

Sehnert, Keith W., *How to be Your Own Doctor—Sometimes*. Grosset & Dunlap, 1975.

Strauss, Maurice B., ed., *Familiar Medical Quotations*. Little, Brown, 1968.

Stuart-Harris, Sir Charles H., and Geoffrey C. Schild, *Influenza: The Viruses and the Disease*. Publishing Sciences Group, 1976.

Swiss Serum and Vaccine Institute, Bern, *Advances in Vaccination against Virus Diseases*. S. Karger, Basil, 1979.

Tan, Leong T., Margaret Y.-C. Tan and Ilza Veith, *Acupuncture Therapy: Current Chinese Practice*. 2nd ed. Temple University Press, 1976.

Thaler, Malcolm S., Richard D. Klausner and Harvey Jay Cohen, eds., *Medical Immunology*. Lippincott, 1977.

Tyrrell, D.A.J. *Common Colds and Related Diseases*. Edward Arnold, 1965.

U.S. Department of Health, Education and Welfare:
*Current Estimates from the Health Interview Survey: United States-1978*. National Center for Health Statistics/Public Health Service, 1979.
*Virology: NIAID Task Force Report*. National Institutes of Health/Public Health Service, 1979.

United States Pharmacopeial Convention, Inc., *United States*. 1980.

Vickery, Donald M., and James F. Fries, *Take Care of Yourself: A Consumer's Guide to Medical Care*. Addison-Wesley, 1976.

Whitney, Eleanor Noss, and Eva May Nunnelley Hamilton, *Understanding Nutrition.* West Publishing, 1977.
Wolf, Stewart, and Helen Goodell, eds., *Harold G. Wolff's Stress and Disease.* Thomas, 1968.
Ziment, Irwin, *Respiratory Pharmacology and Therapeutics.* Saunders, 1978.

**PERIODICALS**
Anderson, Terence W., et al.:
"The Effect on Winter Illness of Large Doses of Vitamin C." *Canadian Medical Association Journal,* Vol. III, July 6, 1974.
"Vitamin C and the Common Cold: A Double-Blind Trial." *Canadian Medical Association Journal,* Vol. 107, Sept. 23, 1972.
"Winter Illness and Vitamin C: The Effect of Relatively Low Doses." *Canadian Medical Association Journal,* Vol. 112, April 5, 1975.
"Aspirin: New Uses for an Old Drug." *Medical World News,* Aug. 6, 1979.
Buckland, et al., "Experiments on the Spread of Colds." *Journal of Hygiene,* Vol. 63, March 1965.
Collis, Peter B., et al., "Adenovirus Vaccines in Military Recruit Populations: A Cost-Benefit Analysis." *The Journal of Infectious Diseases,* Vol. 128, Dec. 1973.
"The Common Cold is Mainly in the Mind." *New Scientist,* Vol. 85, Feb. 1980.
Coulehan, John L., "Ascorbic Acid and the Common Cold." *Postgraduate Medicine,* Vol. 66, Sept. 1979.
D'Alessio, Donn J., et al., "Transmission of Experimental Rhinovirus Colds in Volunteer Married Couples." *The Journal of Infectious Diseases,* Vol. 133, Jan. 1976.
Dowling, Harry F., et al., "Transmission of the Experimental Common Cold in Volunteers." *Journal of Laboratory and Clinical Medicine,* Vol. 50, 1957.
Dykes, Michael H. M., and Paul Meier, "Ascorbic Acid and the Common Cold." *Journal of the American Medical Association,* Vol. 231, March 10, 1975.
Evans, Alfred S., et al., "Acute Respiratory Disease in University of the Philippines and University of Wisconsin Students." *World Health Organization Bulletin,* Vol. 36, 1967.
Gwaltney, Jack M., Jr., et al.:
"Hand-to-Hand Transmission of Rhinovirus Colds." *Annals of Internal Medicine,* Vol. 88, April 1978.
"Rhinovirus Infections in an Industrial Population." *Journal of the American Medical Association,* Vol. 202, Nov. 6, 1967.
"Rhinovirus Transmission—One if by Air, Two if by Hand." *American Journal of Epidemiology,* Vol. 107, May 1978.
Hendley, J. Owen, et al., "Transmission of Rhinovirus Colds by Self-Inoculation." *The New England Journal of Medicine,* Vol. 288, June 28, 1973.
Hirsch, Martin S., et al., "Antiviral Agents." *The New England Journal of Medicine,* Vol. 302, 1980.
Jackson, George Gee, et al., "Transmission of the Common Cold to Volunteers under Controlled Conditions." *AMA Archives of Internal Medicine,* Vol. 101, 1958.
Jackson, George Gee, et al., "Susceptibility and Immunity to Common Upper Respiratory Viral Infections—The Common Cold." *Annals of Internal Medicine,* Vol. 53, 1960.
Kaplan, Martin M., and Robert G. Webster, "The Epidemiology of Influenza." *Scientific American,* Dec. 1977.
Karlowski, Thomas R., et al., "Ascorbic Acid for the Common Cold." *Journal of the American Medical Association,* Vol. 231, March 10, 1975.
"A Leisurely Look at Stress." *The Harvard Medical School Health Letter,* Vol. 4, Oct. 1979.
Manzella, John P., and Norbert J. Roberts Jr., "Human Macrophage and Lymphocyte Responses to Mitogen Stimulation after Exposure to Influenza Virus, Ascorbic Acid, and Hyperthermia." *The Journal of Immunology,* Vol. 123, Nov. 1979.
Marx, Jean L., "Interferon (II): Learning About How It Works." *Science,* Vol. 204, June 22, 1979.
Maugh, Thomas H., II, "Panel Urges Wide Use of Antiviral Drug." *Science,* Vol. 206, Nov. 30, 1979.
Merigan, Thomas C., et al., "Inhibition of Respiratory Virus Infection by Locally Applied Interferon." *The Lancet, I,* March 17, 1973.
Monto, A. S., and H. Ross, "Acute Respiratory Illness in the Community: Effect of Family Composition, Smoking, and Chronic Symptoms." *British Journal of Preventive & Social Medicine,* Vol. 31, June, 1977.
Monto, Arnold S., and Betty M. Ullman, "Acute Respiratory Illness in an American Community: The Tecumseh Study." *Journal of the American Medical Association,* Vol. 227, Jan. 14, 1974.
Muchmore, Harold G., et al., "Respiratory Virus Shedding throughout Isolation at South Pole." *Antarctic Journal, U.S.,* Vol. 14, Oct. 5, 1979.
Proctor, Donald F., "The Upper Airways." *American Review of Respiratory Disease,* Vol. 115, 1977.
Roberts, Norbert J., Jr., "Temperature and Host Defense." *Microbiological Reviews,* Vol. 43, June 1979.
Saketkhoo, Kiumars, et al., "Effects of Drinking Hot Water, Cold Water, and Chicken Soup on Nasal Mucus Velocity and Nasal Airflow Resistance." *CHEST,* Vol. 74, Oct. 1978.
Schmitt, Barton D., *"Fever Phobia." American Journal of Diseases of Children.* Vol. 134, Feb. 1980.
Scoggin, Charles H., and Steven A. Sahn, "The Common Cold—A Few New Tricks That Make the Going Easier." *Modern Medicine,* Vol. 48, Jan. 15-30, 1980.
Sissons, J.G.P., and Michael B. A. Oldstone, "Killing of Virus-Infected Cells by Cytotoxic Lymphocytes." *Journal of Infectious Diseases,* Vol. 142, July 1980.
Smith, Wilson, et al., "A Virus Obtained from Influenza Patients." *The Lancet II,* July 8, 1933.
Stanley, Edith D., et al., "Increased Virus Shedding with Aspirin Treatment of Rhinovirus Infection." *Journal of the American Medical Association,* Vol. 231 March 24, 1975.
Totman, Richard, et al., "Predicting Experimental Colds in Volunteers from Different Measures of Recent Life Stress." *Journal of Psychosomatic Research,* Vol. 24, Nov. 1980.
U.S. Department of Health, Education, and Welfare:
"Amantadine: Does it Have a Role in the Prevention and Treatment of Influenza?" *NIH Consensus Development Conference Summary,* Vol. 2, 1979.
"The Common Cold: Relief But No Cure." *FDA Consumer,* Sept. 1976.
"Influenza Vaccine 1980-81." *Morbidity and Mortality Weekly Report,* Vol. 29, May 16, 1980.
"Over-the-Counter Drugs." *Federal Register,* Part II, Sept. 9, 1976.
Wanner, Adam, "Clinical Aspects of Mucociliary Transport." *American Review of Respiratory Disease,* Vol. 116, 1977.
Weil, Arthur, "33rd Annual Consumer Expenditure Study." *Product Marketing,* Vol. 9, July 1980.

# Picture Credits

*The sources for the illustrations that appear in this book are listed below. Credits for the illustrations from left to right are separated by semicolons, from top to bottom by dashes.*

Cover: Richard Jeffery. 7: National Library of Medicine. 8: Walter E. Hilmers Jr. from HJ Commercial Art. 10: Fil Hunter. 13-16: Trudy Nicholson. 18, 19: Jane Gordon. 20: Erskine L. Palmer from the Electron Microscopy Lab, Center for Disease Control—Bruce D. Korant from Dupont Co.; Merck, Sharp and Dohme Research Laboratories. 21: John L. Gerin from Georgetown University; Dr. J. D. Almeida from Wellcome Research Laboratory, Kent, England—Erskine L. Palmer from the Electron Microscopy Lab, Center for Disease Control; R. C. Valentine from the National Institute for Medical Research, London; Erskine L. Palmer from the Electron Microscopy Lab, Center for Disease Control. 24, 25: Dimis Argyropoulos, Athens. 26, 27: Nathan Benn. 28-31: Ira Block from Woodfin Camp, Inc. 32-35: Loh Wen Kai, courtesy The Chinese Medical Training Institution, Kuala Lumpur. 37: UPI. 39: From *Colds, Coughs, and Catarrh,* by Bernarr Macfadden, Macfadden Publications, Inc., 1926. 40: K. R. Dumbell, London. 41: Jane Gordon. 42: Sankei Shimbun, Tokyo. 44: Imperial War Museum, London. 46: From *Tissues and Organs: A Text-Atlas of Scanning Electron Microscopy,* by Richard G. Kessel and Randy H. Kardon, published by W. H. Freeman and Company, 1979. 47: J. Chao and J. M. Sturgess from the Hospital for Sick Children, Toronto. 48: Fil Hunter, except temperature bar. 50: From *The Breath of Life,* by George Catlin, John Wiley, N.Y., 1861. 52: Walter Reed Army Institute of Research. 54: Dr. Robert Dourmashkin, Clinical Research Center, Middlesex, England. 56: From *Tissues and Organs: A Text-Atlas of Scanning Electron Microscopy,* by Richard G. Kessel and Randy H. Kardon, published by W. H. Freeman and Company, 1979. 57: Bertram Schnitzer, M.D., M. L. Mead, Gregg Gorrin, M.S. from the Department of Pathology at the University of Michigan. 58: Bruce Wetzel, E. Alexander, E. Westbrook from National Cancer Institute. 59: Courtesy Daniel Zagury, Université Pierre et Marie Curie, Paris. 60: *Medical Immunology,* by Malcolm S. Thaler, M.D., Richard D. Klausner, M.D. and Harvey J. Cohen, M.D., J. P. Lippincott & Company, 1977. 63: The Bettmann Archive. 64: Rothco Cartoons, Inc. 65: San Diego, California, Children's Hospital and Health Center. 66: Walter E. Hilmers Jr.

from HJ Commercial Art. 68: Electron Microscopy Staff, D.B.B., Bureau of Biologics, FDA. 71-73: Henry Beville, courtesy the Smithsonian Institution, National Museum of American History. 77: Walter E. Hilmers Jr. from HJ Commercial Art. 79-81: Brian Seed, courtesy The University of Wisconsin at Stevens Point. 83: Jane Gordon. 84: Walter E. Hilmers Jr. from HJ Commercial Art. 86-95: Fil Hunter. 97: Courtesy of Wyeth Laboratories. 99: Walter E. Hilmers Jr. from HJ Commercial Art. 100: Kyoto Shimbun, Kyoto. 102: The Bettmann Archive. 103-107: Walter E. Hilmers Jr. from HJ Commerical Art. 108, 109: Joan S. McGurren. 111: Great, Inc. 113-115: Dorothy Larimer, Director of Public Relations, Oakland, California, Children's Hospital Medical Center. 118, 119: Frederic F. Bigio from B-C Graphics. 122: UPI—Neal Boenzi from The New York Times Pictures. 124, 125: National Archives No. 111-SC-52182. 126, 127: National Archives Nos. 165-WW-269G-3/269G-4. 128, 129: National Archives Nos. 165-WW-269G-6/269G-36/269G-1. 130, 131: National Archives No. 165-WW-269G-8. 132, 133: National Archives Nos. 111-SC-42453, 165-WW-269G-19. 134, 135: National Archives No. 111-SC-153067. 137: © Linda Bartlett 1980. 139: Stanford University. 140: Cartoon by Gilbert Wilkinson, courtesy The Common Cold Unit, Salisbury, England. 142: Cartoon by Arthur Horner, courtesy The Common Cold Unit, Salisbury, England. 144, 145: Lieut. (jg.) Charles C. Curtis, USN Photographic Officer, Naval M. C. Lanyon, New Zealand Support Force, Antarctica. 147: John M. Quarles from Texas A&M University. 149: Wide World. 150: Texas A&M Univeristy. 152-163: Mark Edwards, courtesy MRC, The Common Cold Unit, Salisbury, England.

# Acknowledgments

The index for this book was prepared by Barbara L. Klein. For their valuable help in the preparation of this volume, the editors wish to thank the following: Dr. David W. Alling, National Institute of Allergy and Infectious Diseases, Bethesda, Md.; Terence W. Anderson, University of British Columbia, Vancouver, Canada; Sir Christopher Andrewes, M.D., Salisbury, England; Margaret Andrews, Common Cold Unit, Salisbury, England; Dr. Fakry Assaad, World Health Organization, Geneva, Switzerland; Barbara Aymar, Darien, Conn.; Col. William H. Bancroft, Walter Reed Army Institute of Research, Washington, D.C.; Dr. Samuel Baron, The University of Texas Medical Branch, Galveston, Tex.; Dr. A. S. Beare, Common Cold Unit, Salisbury, England; Dr. Joseph A. Bellanti, Georgetown University School of Medicine, Washington, D.C.; Barbara Berni, American Institute of Acupuncture, Hillsborough, Calif.; Dr. John Betinis, University of Wisconsin-Stevens Point, Wis.; Dr. James Bosma, National Institute of Dental Research, Bethesda, Md.; Victoria Bowling, Ferrum, Va.; Dr. George Cavros, Norfolk, Va.; Judge Tibo J. Chavez, Los Lunas, N. Mex.; Rudolf A. Clemen Jr., American Red Cross National Headquarters, Washington, D.C.; The Clock Hutt, Ltd., New York, N.Y.; Paul Cohen, *Product Marketing,* New York, N.Y.; Dr. Robert Couch, Baylor College of Medicine, Houston, Tex.; Dr. John Coulehan, University of Pittsburgh School of Medicine, Pittsburgh, Pa.; Kathy Cranor, Blacksburg, Va.; Deborah Custer, Kent, Conn.; Dr. Mark Dahl, University of Minnesota Hospital, Minneapolis, Minn.; David Davis, National Reye's Syndrome Foundation, Greater Cincinnati Chapter, Cincinnati, Ohio; Dr. F. W. Davison, Danville, Pa.; Elliot C. Dick, University of Wisconsin Medical School, Madison; Walter R. Dowdle, Centers for Disease Control, Atlanta, Ga.; Dr. David Fairbanks, McLean, Va.; Dr. Bruce Feldman, Chevy Chase, Md.; Dr. Robert Fink, Children's Hospital National Medical Center, Washington, D.C.; S. Fischer, Signature Settings, New York, N.Y.; Dr. Margaret Fletcher, Columbia Medical Plan, Columbia, Md.; Dr. John P. Fox, University of Washington, Seattle; Robert Frank, National Commission on Air Quality, Washington, D.C.; Dr. Robert Friedman, National Institute of Arthritis, Metabolism, and Digestive Diseases, Bethesda, Md.; Joseph R. Geraci, Ontario Veterinary College, Guelph, Canada; Gary Getto, Becton Dickinson Consumer Products, Rochelle Park, N.J.; Dr. Allen Glasgow, Children's Hospital National Medical Center, Washington, D.C.; Dr. Stephen B. Greenberg, Baylor College of Medicine, Houston, Tex.; George B. Griffenhagen, American Pharmaceutical Association, Washington, D.C.; Dr. Jack M. Gwaltney, University of Virginia School of Medicine, Charlottesville; Philip D. Hansten, Washington State University, Pullman; Michael Harris, National Museum of American History, Washington, D.C.; William F. Helfand, Merck, Sharp and Dohme, Rahway, N.J.; John Hierholzer, Centers for Disease Control, Atlanta, Ga.; Dr. Martin S. Hirsch,

Massachusetts General Hospital, Boston; Harrison Hoppes, Flow Laboratories, Inc., McLean, Va.; Dr. Kun-Yen Huang, George Washington University School of Medicine, Washington, D.C.; Everett Jackson, National Museum of American History, Washington, D.C.; Julius A. Kasel, Baylor College of Medicine, Houston, Tex.; Liz Kay, New England Aquarium, Boston, Mass.; James A. Kegel, U.S. Military History Institute, Carlisle Barracks, Pa.; Lucy Keister, National Library of Medicine, Bethesda, Md.; Alan Kendal, Centers for Disease Control, Atlanta, Ga.; Richard G. Kessel, The University of Iowa, Iowa City; Dr. Matthew J. Kluger, University of Michigan Medical School, Ann Arbor; Nan Knight, National Museum of American History, Washington, D.C.; Dr. Vernon Knight, Baylor College of Medicine, Houston, Tex.; John R. La Montagne, National Institute of Allergy and Infectious Diseases, Bethesda, Md.; Dr. David E. Leith, Harvard University School of Public Health, Boston, Mass.; Walter H. Lewis, Washington University, St. Louis, Mo.; Linlo House, New York, N.Y.; John and Pat Lloyd, Worcester, England; John McGinty, University of Connecticut Health Center, Farmington;

Yvonne McHarg, New York, N.Y.; Dr. Richard Marsella, Walter Reed Army Medical Center, Washington, D.C.; Alan W. Mercil, Proprietary Association, Washington, D.C.; Dr. Thomas C. Merigan, Stanford University School of Medicine, Calif.; Dr. Arnold S. Monto, University of Michigan, Ann Arbor; Dr. Harold G. Muchmore, University of Oklahoma, Oklahoma City; George Murakami, New York, N.Y.; Dr. André Nahmias, Emory University School of Medicine, Atlanta, Ga.; Wilton Nichols, Ferrum, Va.; Richard Penna, American Pharmaceutical Association, Washington, D.C.; Stephen M. Peters, Georgetown University Medical Center, Washington, D.C.; James C. Pettersen, University of Wisconsin, Madison; Ella R. Pfeiffer, Arlington, Va.; Dr. Donald F. Proctor, The Johns Hopkins University School of Hygiene and Public Health, Baltimore, Md.; John M. Quarles, Texas A&M University, College Station; Dr. Gerald V. Quinnan Jr., Food and Drug Administration, Rockville, Md.; Dr. Sylvia E. Reed, Public Health Laboratory Service, London, England; Dr. Norbert J. Roberts, University of Rochester School of Medicine, N.Y.; Robert Schreiber, National Institute of Allergy and Infectious Diseases,

Bethesda, Md.; Dr. Jerome L. Schulman, Mount Sinai School of Medicine of the City University of New York, N.Y.; Arthur Silverstein, The Johns Hopkins Hospital, Baltimore, Md.; Dorothy Smith, American Pharmaceutical Association, Washington, D.C.; Mr. and Mrs. Jessie E. Smith, Stockton, Calif.; Ruth Smith, London House, Arlington, Va.; Sir Charles Stuart-Harris, M.D., University of Sheffield Medical School, England; David C. Swift, The Johns Hopkins University School of Hygiene and Public Health, Baltimore, Md.; Sue Thiemann, University of California, San Francisco, Calif.; K. R. Thompson, Common Cold Unit, Salisbury, England; Eddie Tso, Navajo Health Authority, Window Box, Ariz.; Duane Voth, New York, N.Y.; Peggy Wakefield, Children's Hospital Medical Center of Northern California, Oakland; Dr. John Wallace, Common Cold Unit, Salisbury, England; Dr. Adam Wanner, Mount Sinai Medical Center, Miami Beach, Fla.; Dr. Peter A. Ward, University of Michigan Medical School, Ann Arbor; Manfred Waserman, National Library of Medicine, Bethesda, Md.; Arthur Weil, *Product Marketing,* New York, N.Y.; Wu Jing-Nuan, Washington, D.C.

# Index *Numerals in italics indicate an illustration of the subject mentioned.*